OVERCOMING PROCRASTINATION

WINDY DRYDEN was born in London in 1950. He has worked in psychotherapy and counselling for over twenty-five years, and is the author or editor of over 100 books, including *Ten Steps to Positive Living* (Sheldon Press, 1994) and *How to Accept Yourself* (Sheldon Press, 1999). Dr Dryden is Professor of Counselling at Goldsmiths College, University of London.

Overcoming Common Problems Series

For a full list of titles please contact
Sheldon Press, Marylebone Road, London NW1 4DU

Overcoming Common Problems Series

Overcoming Common Problems Series

Overcoming Common Problems

Overcoming Procrastination

Dr Windy Dryden

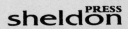

First published in Great Britain in 2000 by
Sheldon Press, SPCK,
Holy Trinity Church, Marylebone Road, London NW1 4DU

British Library Cataloguing-in-Publication Data

A catalogue record for this book is available from the British Library

ISBN 0–85969–815–7

Typeset by Deltatype Limited, Birkenhead, Merseyside
Printed in Great Britain by
Biddles Ltd, Guildford and King's Lynn

Contents

Preface

I have never really suffered from procrastination. If anything, I try to do tasks well before their deadline. Does this qualify me to write a book on overcoming procrastination? I think it does. You may think that it would be better if I used to procrastinate but learned to overcome it – and you may be right. However, this is not the case. I bring to this book my knowledge of why people procrastinate and what can be done to help them, my own experience as a counsellor of helping people to overcome their procrastination problems over twenty-five years, and my experience of living a life when it comes to doing things on – and in most instances ahead of – time.

I have divided this book into three parts. In Part 1, I consider the nature of procrastination, why we do it and how we can overcome it in general terms. In Part 2, I consider the different specific types of procrastination and how to deal with each specific type. You will only get most out of this material if you have digested and practised the material in Part 1. Finally, in Part 3, I outline a smorgasbord of practical and psychological tips to overcome procrastination.

Throughout the book, I stress the importance of identifying, challenging and changing the unhealthy beliefs that underpin all forms of procrastination and the importance of developing an anti-procrastination philosophy. You may be tempted to go straight to Part 3 of the book to discover quick and easy ways of overcoming your procrastination problems. Resist this temptation. Again, you need to digest and implement the material in Part 1 of the book before the advice that I give in Part 3 will have any lasting impact.

There is no quick fix answer to overcoming procrastination. That's the bad news. The good news is that you can help yourself enormously by applying and applying again the methods that I outline (particularly in Part 1). So, don't just read this book. Use it! If you do, you may be pleasantly surprised with the results.

Windy Dryden

PART 1

Procrastination: What it is, Why You do it and What You Can Do About it

1
What is Procrastination?

A recent consumer report on the amount of time we in Britain squander makes alarming reading. The report showed that we spend on average each week: 1 hour 30 minutes stuck in traffic jams, 36 minutes waiting for public transport, 1 hour 24 minutes dealing with bureaucracy, 1 hour 12 minutes waiting in queues at shops or banks, 1 hour 24 minutes looking for things at home, 1 hour 18 minutes shopping for things without success. All in all we squander about seven and a half hours each week in the above ways, which approximates to about two and a half years over the average lifetime.

While we may not have much control over some of these factors, we do have much more control over how we spend our time in other areas. But do we use this time wisely? Do we do tasks that are in our interests to do when it is in our interests to do them? The answer is that some of us do, but most of us don't. Most of us procrastinate. What does the term 'procrastination' mean? It means putting off until tomorrow what is in our interests to do today. Thus procrastination has three major features:

- a task that it is in our interests to do;
- a time frame in which it is important for us to take action;
- a postponement of this action until another time.

In addition, procrastination involves one or more additional postponements until action is taken:

- either at the very last minute;
- after the due deadline;
- action is not taken at all.

We all procrastinate at some time in our lives. How many of us, for example, have not put off paying a bill until the very last moment when it would have been better for us to pay it earlier? It is certainly not my intention to write a book hoping to persuade you to banish all forms of procrastination from your life. If this was my intention then I would

3

inevitably fail. No, I have written this book mainly for those who have a chronic problem with procrastination and who suffer needlessly from routinely putting things off in one or a number of areas in their lives.

Major procrastination areas

Before I discuss chronic procrastination more fully, let me briefly review the basic areas in which we procrastinate. In the field of human endeavour it is possible to procrastinate over anything at all, but it seems to me and others who have written on the subject that we procrastinate in the areas of:

- personal maintenance;
- self-development;
- honouring commitments to others.

While these three areas can and often do overlap, I will deal with each area briefly in turn.

Personal maintenance

When we procrastinate in the area of personal maintenance we put off taking action that will maintain our lives in the following areas: health, personal cleanliness, finance, personal administration, general living conditions (such as cleaning, organizing and maintaining our living quarters) and work.

Self-development

When we procrastinate in the area of self-development we put off taking action that will enhance our lives in a variety of areas, such as: developing personal interests, improving opportunities for advancement in our chosen line of work, gaining further educational qualifications and broadening knowledge in specific and/or general areas.

Honouring commitments to others

Sometimes we make commitments to others which at the time we are fully prepared to honour, but which later we regret making or regard as onerous. Instead of 'biting the bullet' and doing whatever we agreed to for other people, we put off doing it, hoping perhaps that the other person will have forgotten the promise that we made to them. For example, I have edited a number of academic texts and I usually give those who agree to contribute a very generous amount of time to complete their chapter. However, a number of my contributors submit their chapters late, thus inconveniencing both me as editor and the publishers, who usually have tight publication schedules.

Having covered the main areas in which we procrastinate, let me discuss the nature of chronic procrastination in greater detail.

Chronic procrastination: when things really get bad

As I have already stated, this book is mainly for people who have chronic procrastination. As I alluded to above, there are two types of chronic procrastination:

* chronic specific procrastination;
* chronic general procrastination.

If you have chronic specific procrastination, you tend to have a long-standing problem doing things on time in one area of your life, but in other areas of your life you do not have a problem with procrastination. Thus, one of my clients does things on time and often well before time in all areas of her life except one. She procrastinates on tasks that have anything to do with her tax affairs and has done so for years. This has resulted in numerous fines and time-consuming audits, none of which would have happened had she dealt with her tax affairs on time.

If you have chronic general procrastination, you tend to procrastinate in a number of important areas in your life, you have tended to do so for years and you routinely suffer from doing so. It perhaps goes without saying that chronic procrastination is difficult to overcome, and this is particularly so when you have chronic general procrastination because it has almost become a way of life for you.

Help is at hand

I have two pieces of good news and one piece of bad news for you. The first piece of good news is that you can help yourself to overcome both types of chronic procrastination. I have helped hundreds of people whose lives have been blighted by their avoidant style of dealing with issues that were better confronted to overcome their procrastination problem.

The bad news is that you will not find this easy to do. Before you close this book and put it aside (which if you have a chronic problem with procrastination you will be strongly tempted to do at this point), please give me a chance to explain.

Chronic procrastination is by definition a bad habit, and habits take time to break. There is no getting around this grim fact. However, if you accept this point (without necessarily liking it), you will at least give yourself a chance to break your bad procrastinating habit. All you need to have is the following:

- *Awareness* – that you are in fact procrastinating.
- *Goal-directedness* – a wish to do the task that you are currently avoiding (or a wish to have the task done).
- *Commitment* – to put up with short-term pains for longer-term gains.
- *Persistence* – a willingness to repeat the procedures that I will discuss throughout the book until they become second nature to you.

Now, if you have chronic procrastination (either in a specific area or more generally), you may think that you are particularly deficient in the above qualities unless they are in the service of procrastination. Thus, you may be only too aware that you are procrastinating and that your goal is to avoid doing difficult, threatening or aversive tasks. You may well acknowledge that you have committed yourself to procrastination and are very persistent at continuing to actively avoid these tasks that are in your interests to do.

My point is that you do have the skills of awareness, setting goals, committing yourself to a course of action and being persistent (albeit at continuing to put things off). I don't need to teach you these skills: you have them already and are pretty good at using them. What I want to encourage you to do is to use those skills in areas where they help you rather than hinder you as at present. This is my second piece of good news for you: I do not have to teach you things that you are not good at; all I need to do is to encourage you to transfer these skills to areas that will help you live a more effective, satisfying life than one based on avoidance and self-deception.

I hope I have at least interested you enough for you to continue to read this book. As I have said, the road to overcoming procrastination is not easy, but it can be done and, as I have just shown you, you have all the tools at your disposal to help you to make this difficult but rewarding journey.

2
How to Tell if You are Procrastinating

If you suffer from chronic specific procrastination, and particularly if your chronic procrastination problem is more general in nature, you are probably very adept at deceiving yourself. You probably have a number of rationalizations and plausible excuses up your sleeve that you tell yourself at the drop of a hat to explain why, in fact, you are not procrastinating. So how do you tell if you are procrastinating? In order to answer this question you need to be straight with yourself. Ask yourself a number of questions and, having done so, come up with honest answers to these questions. The first question is as follows:

Is it in my best interests to do this task?

If it is not in your best interests to do the task in question, then you are not procrastinating when you put it off. It may be that someone else wants you to do the task for their own reasons or that the other person may think that it is in your best interests to do it. However, none of these factors necessarily means that doing the task serves a good purpose for *you*. So come up with good reasons why it is in your best interests to do the task. If you are in two minds about this do a cost-benefit analysis on the issue.

When you do a cost-benefit analysis you specify two options, one which involves doing the task and the other which involves not doing it. You then specify which of your best interests you think the activity is designed to meet. Let me provide an illustration from my own life. My choice is whether I should exercise or not. Thus I have two options:

Option 1 Swimming for 30 minutes a day.
Option 2 Lying in bed instead of going swimming.

Then, I specify which of my best interests I think swimming will serve:

Best interests served Maintaining my health.

Table 1 provides a cost-benefit analysis form which I suggest that you use to answer the question: Is it in my best interests to do the task? You will note that the form has three major components. First, it asks you to

7

consider the advantages (or benefits) and the disadvantages (or costs) that accrue to each option. Second, it asks you to consider these advantages both from a short-term perspective and from a long-term perspective, and finally, it asks you to consider these advantages and disadvantages as they accrue to yourself and to others who are involved. Keep your best interests clearly in mind when deciding which option to choose.

Table 1 Cost-benefit analysis form

ADVANTAGES/BENEFITS OF _____

SHORT TERM
For yourself   For other people

1:   1:

2:   2:

3:   3:

4:   4:

5:   5:

6:   6:

LONG TERM
For yourself   For other people

1:   1:

2:   2:

3:   3:

4:   4:

5:   5:

6:   6:

DISADVANTAGES/COSTS OF

SHORT TERM

For yourself	For other people
1:	1:
2:	2:
3:	3:
4:	4:
5:	5:
6:	6:

LONG TERM

For yourself	For other people
1:	1:
2:	2:
3:	3:
4:	4:
5:	5:
6:	6:

ADVANTAGES/BENEFITS OF

SHORT TERM

For yourself	For other people
1:	1:

2:                              2:

3:                              3:

4:                              4:

5:                              5:

6:                              6:

LONG TERM
For yourself   For other people

1:                              1:

2:                              2:

3:                              3:

4:                              4:

5:                              5:

6:                              6:

DISADVANTAGES/COSTS OF

SHORT TERM
For yourself   For other people

1:                              1:

2:                              2:

3:                              3:

4:                              4:

5:                              5:

6:                              6:

LONG TERM
For yourself   For other people

1:                              1:

2:                              2:

3:                              3:

4:                              4:

5:                              5:

6:                              6:

Table 2 shows the cost-benefit analysis that I did on whether I should get up early to exercise or lie in bed. You will note that there appears to be more in favour of my lying in bed in the morning in the short term than of getting up to exercise, whereas the picture clearly favours the swimming option when the longer term is considered. So why do I decide to swim? Because it is in the best interests of my continuing health to do so.

Table 2 Example of a completed cost-benefit analysis form

ADVANTAGES/BENEFITS OF Swimming for 30 minutes a day

SHORT TERM
For yourself   For other people

1:                              1:

2:                              2:

3:                              3:

4:                                    4:

5:                                    5:

6:                                    6:

LONG TERM

For yourself   For other people

1: Swimming is good for my   1:
   back

2: Swimming is good overall   2:
   exercise

3: Regular swimming gives me   3:
   increased energy

4: Regular swimming gives me a   4:
   greater sense of well-being

5:                                    5:

6:                                    6:

DISADVANTAGES/COSTS OF Swimming for 30 minutes a day

SHORT TERM

For yourself   For other people

1: I experience discomfort by   1: Getting up early wakes up my
   getting up early   wife

2: I lose out on an extra 30   2:
   minutes' rest

3: I miss out on listening to the   3:
   news on the radio

4:	4:
5:	5:
6:	6:

LONG TERM

For yourself	For other people
1: I lose out on the benefits of 30 minutes' extra rest a day	1: Wife may be more tired if I regularly wake her up early
2:	2:
3:	3:
4:	4:
5:	5:
6:	6:

ADVANTAGES/BENEFITS OF Lying in bed instead of going swimming

SHORT TERM

For yourself	For other people
1: Get an extra 30 minutes' rest	1: Don't disturb my wife by getting up early
2: Remain comfortable	2:
3: Stay in the warm	3:
4: Can listen to the radio if I want to	4:

5:                                    5:

6:                                    6:

LONG TERM
For yourself   For other people

1: May benefit from extra 30   1: Wife may benefit by not being
   minutes' rest a day   disturbed by my getting up
                                         early

2:                                    2:

3:                                    3:

4:                                    4:

5:                                    5:

6:                                    6:

DISADVANTAGES/COSTS OF Lying in bed instead of going swimming

SHORT TERM
For yourself   For other people

1:                                    1:

2:                                    2:

3:                                    3:

4:                                    4:

5:                                    5:

6:                                    6:

LONG TERM

For yourself

For other people

1: Miss out on regular exercise
1:

2: Decreased energy
2:

3: More lower back pain
3:

4: Miss out on my greater sense
of well-being that regular
swimming gives me
4:

5:
5:

6:
6:

This points to a central issue in understanding the dynamics of procrastination. It is so important that I am going to put it in a box so that it stands out for you.

> People procrastinate when they routinely give more weight to the short-term advantages of avoiding doing what is in their best interests to do than to the longer-term advantages of doing the task concerned.

So when you consider whether or not the task under consideration is in your best interests, consider the longer-term issues as well as the short-term issues. If you are still in doubt, ask yourself what advice you would give a close friend or relative who provided you with the same information on the cost-benefit analysis form as you came up with yourself. Thus, if I was in two minds about swimming over lying in bed and a close friend asked me what he should do in the same circumstances, I would clearly advise him to go swimming if he was concerned to maintain his health.

When is it in my best interests to do the task?

Having ascertained that it is in your best interests to do the task, the next step is for you to determine when you are going to take action. If you suffer from chronic specific procrastination, however, you will still easily put off doing something that you know in your heart of hearts is in your best interests to do. If asked, you can come up with a whole host of reasons why it's better to start tomorrow than to begin today. Thus, the second question to ask yourself to which it is advisable to respond with complete candour concerns *when* it is in your best interests to take action.

Often the most appropriate answer to this question is straight away, although in this busy world of ours, where we have many things to do, it isn't always realistic to do something immediately. Thus, it is wise to develop a timetable to help you to decide what you are going to do and when you are going to do it. This is particularly useful when it is in your interests to repeat the same action several times a week, perhaps at different times, like an exercise regime. For example, in my own case, my chosen swimming regime involves going to the pool five days a week and swimming for 30 minutes per day. In addition, I specify in advance which days of the week I will go swimming and at what time I need to leave the house so that I can best fit my swimming sessions into my daily schedule. I thus have a very clear and specific note of when it is in my best interests to go swimming, and having such a clear and specific note of when I am going to take action, I know very quickly when I am beginning to procrastinate. And if I do begin to procrastinate I can take immediate steps to remedy the situation and get back on track.

If you do have a chronic problem with procrastination, it is likely that you only have a very vague idea concerning when it is in your best interests to do any particular task. Since your timetable is so loose it is very easy for you to convince yourself that you will begin to take action soon, and for you to postpone making a decision to start by reiterating to yourself that you will begin soon. Of course, 'soon' is so vague that it is always on the horizon and becomes both a comfort ('I will begin soon') and a trap ('soon' may never become 'now').

So if you want to overcome procrastination, it is very important that you set very clear and specific guidelines concerning when you are to begin any given task so that you know immediately when you are beginning to procrastinate. Starting immediately is perhaps the best policy in most cases, but if that is not feasible at least set a very specific starting time.

When is it legitimate to put off taking action?

As I have already mentioned, if you suffer from chronic specific or general procrastination, it is likely that you have developed a real talent for deceiving yourself. Specifically, you probably give yourself numerous reasons why now is not the right time to begin the task that it is in your best interests to do. As I have explained in the previous section, setting a specific start time will help you to know when you are beginning to procrastinate, but you will still develop what seem to you perfectly good reasons to postpone taking action. It is important that you find a way of distinguishing between legitimate and illegitimate reasons for delaying the starting time that you have agreed with yourself. Somebody once joked that the only legitimate reason for postponing an agreed starting time is death! However, there are often less drastic legitimate reasons for postponing your starting time. These legitimate reasons mean that you are sensibly postponing the work that you need to do on the task and that you are, in fact, not procrastinating.

What are legitimate reasons for sensibly postponing taking action on a task? My view is that the following constitute legitimate reasons for postponing action:

Physical illness

If you are ill you may well not have the physical energy or the mental capacity to concentrate on the task at hand. Indeed, if you begin the task when you are ill, you may well make yourself more ill. Thus, if you consider that because of illness you are not in a position to begin a task then it is legitimate for you to postpone taking action until you have recovered.

Emotional disturbance

If you are in a state of emotional disturbance about an issue that does not impinge on the task at hand, then it is unlikely that you will be able to concentrate enough to do the task unless it is quite simple and requires little concentration to complete. Thus, if you are depressed about losing an important relationship and the task that is in your best interests to do is reasonably complex, then, in my opinion, it is legitimate for you to postpone the task until you are over your depression. Conversely, if the task cannot wait until then it is legitimate

- to ask another person to help you with the task;
- to ask that person to do the task for you if that is appropriate;
- to negotiate a new deadline with other involved parties.

Other disturbed emotional states that are legitimate reasons for task postponement include anxiety, unhealthy anger, guilt, shame, unhealthy jealousy, hurt and unhealthy envy. Also, if you are under the influence of alcohol or a drug then it does not make sense for you to tackle the task at hand. If you are experiencing any of these disturbed emotional states then it is important that you deal with them yourself or seek counselling before you tackle the relevant task. If your disturbed emotion relates to the task at hand then again you need to deal with these feelings before you physically tackle the task. Doing so, in fact, is a legitimate way of overcoming procrastination, and I will address this issue throughout this book.

Skills deficiency

It sometimes happens that the task that is in your interests to do calls upon you to use a skill that you may not possess. In such cases, it makes perfect sense for you to delay taking action until you have learned the necessary skill. If, of course, you delay learning this skill, then you are procrastinating.

Ignorance

Sometimes you cannot begin a task that is in your interests to do because you lack an important piece of information that is crucial for you to have before you begin the task. For example, one of my friends decided to repair his lawn mower rather than to send it away for repair, because he needed to save money. He had the requisite skills to repair the lawn mower, but he lost the operating instructions that he needed to do the job properly. His decision to delay beginning the job until he had obtained another copy of the operating instructions was a legitimate reason to postpone the task and was thus not an example of procrastination. Again, however, if my friend had put off obtaining the instructions that he needed to do the task, he would have been procrastinating.

Facing a crisis

The final legitimate reason for postponing beginning a task that is in your best interests to do, at a time that you have agreed with yourself to do it, is when you face a sudden and unexpected crisis in your life. To put this starkly: if you have agreed with yourself to start work on an essay at 9 a.m. on a Friday morning and at 8.55 a.m. you get a call to say that your mother has been taken seriously ill and has been rushed to hospital, then it is clearly not procrastination to put off beginning the essay and to go to the hospital as quickly as possible. Indeed, it would be quite bizarre for you to say to yourself that visiting your mother could wait since you were going to keep your agreement with yourself and begin the essay at 9 a.m.

So there you have it: having decided that a particular task is in your interests to do and having allotted a starting time, I argue that it is legitimate to postpone beginning the task if you are ill, feeling emotionally disturbed about an unrelated issue, discover that you lack the skills or important knowledge to begin the task, or face a sudden and unexpected crisis which requires your full attention to meet. These reasons involve you making a considered decision to delay doing the task under consideration, which is not procrastination. Having a legitimate reason to postpone a task is a characteristic of what is called 'planned delay'. Lacking such a reason is a characteristic of procrastination.

So unless you have one or more of the above reasons for postponing a task, you are probably on safe ground in concluding that you are procrastinating. However, if you suffer from chronic procrastination you will recognize that it is only too easy for you to take what I have listed as legitimate reasons to delay tackling a task and use them to convince yourself that you have a good reason to put off beginning the task when in fact you have no such reason. Such is your talent at self-deceit if you suffer from chronic procrastination.

Thus, you can easily persuade yourself that you are feeling ill or are suffering from diffuse feelings of anxiety. Furthermore, you can easily persuade yourself that you lack a key skill to do a task when in fact you don't, or that you lack crucial information that turns out not to be crucial at all. Finally, you can easily label an event as a crisis when it is no more than a moderate inconvenience. This is why I say that unless you are prepared to be completely candid with yourself and identify, but not be guided by, your habitual attempts to deceive yourself into thinking that you have legitimate reasons for postponing taking appropriate action, then I can assure you that you will continue to suffer from chronic procrastination.

So far you have done the following:

- You have ascertained that it is in your best interests to do a task.
- You have identified when it is in your best interests to do it.
- You have distinguished between legitimate and illegitimate reasons for putting off taking action.

You are now in a position to discover more precisely why you procrastinate. In the next chapter, I will help you to do so by giving an overview of the broad psychological themes that lie behind your procrastination.

3
Understanding the Broad Psychological Themes behind Your Procrastination

In this chapter, I will discuss the major broad psychological themes that lie behind your procrastination. In subsequent chapters, I will deal with each theme in more detail. Understanding the psychological issues that underpin your procrastination is a crucial step because if you don't understand the issue (or issues) that apply to you, you will be disadvantaged in trying to overcome your chronic procrastination. Not that such understanding alone is all you need to overcome your problem. Far from it. I usually put it this way to my clients. Understanding the psychological issues that lie behind your procrastination problem is a necessary step towards overcoming this problem, but it is insufficient to solve the problem. This means that if you don't understand the psychological issues involved you won't overcome your problem, but to overcome it you need more than this understanding. Bear this point in mind as I introduce you to the broad psychological themes that are found in the vast majority of cases of chronic procrastination.

As we have seen, procrastination means putting off until tomorrow what it is in your interests to do today (or at least at a time that you have sensibly set aside to do it). In this chapter I will discuss, in broad terms at first, the main psychological issues that lie behind this 'putting off'.

Procrastination as avoidance

Much of procrastination is an example of what psychologists call avoidance behaviour. I have been a counsellor and psychotherapist for twenty-five years, and in that time I have helped many people from all walks of life tackle their chronic procrastination problem. In doing so, it seems to me that what people are trying to avoid when they procrastinate can be broken down into two main areas. First, we procrastinate because we are trying to avoid something that we find threatening. I call this 'Avoidance of Threat'. Second, we procrastinate because we predict that we will experience discomfort if we face up to the situation. I call this 'Avoidance of Discomfort'.

21

I will discuss these two types of avoidance more fully in future chapters.

Procrastination as restoring the balance

While avoidance-based procrastination is perhaps the most common form of procrastination, other forms of procrastination exist which don't primarily involve threat and discomfort. Thus, some people seem to procrastinate because they view procrastination as restoring some kind of balance in their minds. As we will see later, the psychological issue I have called 'restoring the balance' is clearly found in people whose sense of autonomy is easily threatened. For such people, procrastination is a way of restoring the balance when it comes to their sense of autonomy. Procrastination gives them a sense that they are autonomous individuals who will do tasks when they choose to do them and not when others want them to do them.

Procrastination as prelude

When procrastination occurs purely as a prelude, the person who is procrastinating is not doing so because she is avoiding any kind of threat in her mind, or because she is trying to restore some kind of balance in her mind, or for any other reason apart from her deeply held conviction that she needs to put things off until the last moment when she will galvanize herself into action and come through brilliantly at the death. Although people whose procrastination is a prelude to the final overture of last-minute action do partly acknowledge that they have a problem with procrastination, so addicted are they to last-minute intense activity that they are quite ambivalent about wishing to change. Hence, if you recognize procrastination as prelude as a major feature of your procrastination then I strongly suggest that you do a cost-benefit analysis on when it is best for you to begin a task: either at the last minute or earlier in the process (see pp. 7–15 for details of the cost-benefit analysis method).

Procrastination as an interpersonal ploy

Alfred Adler, a famous psychologist, once said that all behaviour has a purpose. Thus, we have to ask what purpose procrastination serves for you, if we are truly to understand your chronic procrastination. We have already seen that procrastination serves the purpose of helping us to avoid dealing with something that we find threatening or uncomfortable, or that it helps us to restore in our minds some balance in our relationships with others. We have even seen that procrastination serves a purpose as being a prelude to frenzied last-minute task-related activity. However, when procrastination serves a more explicit interpersonal purpose, it is designed to elicit a particular kind of response from others. Now, I want to make clear that this is not necessarily a fully conscious strategy on the part of the person who is procrastinating, although, of course, it can be used with deliberate and fully conscious intent which, however, is concealed from the other person (or people) involved. For example, one of the most common responses that procrastination is designed to elicit from others is for them to take over and do the work for you. While most often you may not be fully aware that this is what you are trying to bring about, sometimes you may be fully aware of it, particularly if it has ceased to be successful!

When procrastination is used (either consciously or sub-consciously) to get others to take over and do the work for you, frequently but not always this is accompanied by you making what appears to be a serious, but obviously (to the other person) hopeless attempt to do the task. I want to make clear that this attempt is part of the procrastination strategy rather than a serious attempt on your behalf to do the task. On witnessing you struggling in an apparently serious but doomed attempt to do the task, the other person's sympathy or concern is elicited and that person offers to do the task for you. When this offer is made, you make a protest (which you sincerely hope is not taken seriously) and when the other person overrides your protest, you allow them to take over with much gratitude. On other occasions, you show the other person that you are quite paralysed with procrastination and cannot be expected to make even a hopelessly doomed attempt to do the task.

For this strategy to work, the other person has to be ignorant of your strategic use of procrastination and they either have to have a personal investment in the task being done or they have to derive a psychological payoff for doing the task for you. Frequently, people who are prepared to take over for you are those who

- experience other-pity and can't bear to see you suffer;
- have a need to be needed;
- derive psychological benefit from playing the role of rescuer.

If you are particularly adept at using procrastination as a ploy to get others to take over for you, you are very effective at choosing the target of your strategy.

Other responses that procrastination is designed to elicit from others include:

- eliciting help from others (this is different from you seeking others to do the work for you, in the sense that you gain comfort from doing the task with someone rather than having the other do it for you);
- getting sympathy from the other person (this is often sufficient for you to do the task);
- gaining another's interest (again this helps you to begin the task at hand);
- provoking anger from the other person (this may either galvanize you into action, with the purpose of showing the other that you can do the task if they angrily accuse you of shirking, for example, or it may give you justification for not doing the task at all).

When procrastination is basically an interpersonal ploy, it is important to ask yourself what response you hope others will give you when they notice you procrastinating. It is even more important that you are completely candid with yourself in answering this question.

Procrastination as logical consequence

When I say that procrastination is a logical consequence, what I mean by this is that it is often the inevitable consequence of an overcommitted life-style. Indeed, if your procrastination directly results from being overcommitted, your real problem isn't really procrastination, for you often do a lot of things on time. However, you put some things off because you have too much on your plate. Your real problem is allowing yourself to be overcommitted, and the main reason why you do this is that you have a problem saying no, for reasons that I will discuss presently.

I have now briefly discussed the five major psychological broad themes that lie behind procrastination. Before leaving this topic, to which I will return later in the book in greater detail, I do wish to stress that while I have dealt with these five broad themes separately, they can occur in combination in any given individual's chronic procrastination problem. Thus, underpinning your problem with chronic procrastina-

24

tion might be the following issues: avoidance of threat, avoidance of discomfort and a ploy to get others to do the task for you. If this is the case, if you are truly to overcome your chronic procrastination, it is important that you deal successfully with all three areas.

4

The Real Reason Why You Procrastinate: Your Beliefs

In the previous chapter, I discussed in broad terms the five major psychological themes that underpin chronic procrastination. I will return to each of these themes in greater detail later, but first I want to deal with the core of this book and what to my mind is the core of why people procrastinate. In this chapter, then, I will outline my view that the main reason why you procrastinate in chronic fashion is that you hold tenaciously to a set of beliefs (or attitudes) that impel you to put off until tomorrow what is in your best interests to do today.

Let me explain more fully what I mean. Let's suppose that the major psychological theme involved in your procrastination is avoidance of discomfort. This means that every time you either feel discomfort or anticipate experiencing discomfort as you approach the task that is in your best interests to do, you put off doing it. The main point I want you to grasp is that it is *not* the experience of discomfort (or its anticipation) on its own that causes you to procrastinate. Rather, your belief or attitude towards the discomfort is the main reason why you put off doing the task.

There are five possible beliefs that you could hold about discomfort about doing the task. Only one explains why you procrastinate. Here are the five beliefs:

Belief A   It is essential that I am uncomfortable when I do a task

If you held this belief you certainly would not procrastinate when you experienced discomfort related to doing the task at hand. Indeed, you would procrastinate if you didn't experience discomfort. The experience of discomfort would be essential before you set about doing the task at hand. So this belief certainly doesn't account for your procrastination. If you experience discomfort while holding Belief A, this belief is known as a met demand.

26

Belief B   It is preferable that I experience discomfort before I do the task at hand. Discomfort isn't essential in this respect, but it is desirable

Again, if you held this belief you would not procrastinate when you experienced discomfort related to the task at hand because you would hope to experience such discomfort before beginning the task. Thus, this belief would also not account for your procrastination. If you experience discomfort while holding Belief B, this belief is known as a met preference.

Belief C   I don't care whether I am comfortable or uncomfortable before I do the task at hand. I'm just not bothered one way or the other. If the task has to be done I will do it no matter whether I experience discomfort or not

This is known as an indifference belief, and again does not really explain why you would procrastinate. Indeed, as you make clear, the issue of experiencing discomfort is not relevant to your procrastination.

Belief D   It is preferable that I experience comfort before I do the task at hand. Comfort isn't essential in this respect, but it is desirable

If you held this belief you would still not procrastinate if you experienced discomfort relating to the task at hand, because you would only deem it undesirable if you felt uncomfortable. This undesirable state would not stop you from doing the task if you were clear that it was in your best interests to do it. For example, whenever I wake up in the morning, I would prefer to stay in bed rather than get up to go swimming. My preference does not stop me from getting up because I am clear that it is in my best interests to go swimming, and as the pool isn't going to come into my bed, I will have to get up and go to it if I am to act in my best interests. If you experience discomfort while holding Belief D, this is known as an unmet preference.

Belief E It is absolutely essential that I am comfortable when I do a task

This is the only belief of the five that I have presented which explains your procrastination when you experience (or anticipate experiencing) discomfort. You are not just putting forward a preference about feeling comfort (as in Belief D), you are making an absolute demand about not starting the task until you are comfortable. Thus, you will procrastinate on the task as long as you experience (or anticipate experiencing) discomfort. If you experience discomfort while holding Belief E, this belief is known as an unmet demand.

To put this slightly differently, when you experience (or anticipate experiencing) discomfort and you hold the unmet preference outlined in Belief D, you still have room for manoeuvre because this belief is flexible (i.e. you state that you prefer to be comfortable before beginning the task at hand, but you do not insist that you have to be comfortable before doing so). Consequently, you give yourself leeway with respect to beginning the task even if you are uncomfortable and thus, holding this belief, you will not procrastinate if you see clearly that the task is worth doing. However, when you experience (or anticipate experiencing) discomfort and you hold the unmet demand outlined above in Belief E, you no longer have room for manoeuvre because this belief is inflexible (i.e. you insist that you have to be comfortable before doing the task). Consequently, you give yourself no leeway with respect to beginning the task when you are uncomfortable and thus, holding this belief, you will procrastinate even if you see clearly that the task is worth doing.

In summary, it is not what you consider to be a threat that causes you to procrastinate, nor does feeling uncomfortable or considering yourself to be in a state of imbalance directly lead you to put off until tomorrow what is wiser for you to do today, to give but three examples. Rather, it is your belief about these events that largely leads you to procrastinate. Furthermore, it is a particular type of belief – a rigid, inflexible demand that certain conditions (e.g. being free from threat, discomfort or imbalance) absolutely must exist before you do the task at hand – that explains why you procrastinate.

The four unhealthy beliefs that explain why you procrastinate

In the previous section, I made the crucial point that the main reason you procrastinate is because you hold a rigid belief, a demand that certain conditions must exist or that other conditions must not exist before you begin to do the task that it is in your best interests to do. Dr Albert Ellis, the famous American clinical psychologist, considers that these rigid beliefs, which often take the form of musts, absolute shoulds, have to's or got to's, are at the very core of procrastination. Dr Ellis, who founded an approach to counselling and psychotherapy known as Rational Emotive Behaviour Therapy (REBT) upon which this book is based, also argues that people whose problem is chronic specific or general procrastination hold three further unhealthy beliefs that explain why they procrastinate.

Before I discuss all four unhealthy beliefs in turn, I want to make two points. First, Dr Ellis argues that rigid demands are at the very core of procrastination and that the three further unhealthy beliefs are derived from these demands. While not all REBT therapists agree with Ellis's position on this point, you should at least consider Ellis's views on the primacy of rigid demands as you learn more about the factors that underpin your own procrastination problem.

Second, while I will discuss four unhealthy beliefs in this section, I do not mean to imply that all four beliefs are always present in all forms of chronic procrastination. Please remember this, because while I want you to identify the unhealthy beliefs that underpin your own procrastination problem I do not want you to own up to holding beliefs that you do not, in fact, hold.

Third, there are three qualities that make unhealthy beliefs unhealthy. First, they are inconsistent with reality, i.e. they are false; second, they do not make logical sense; and finally, they are not helpful (in this context, they lead to procrastination rather than task performance).

Let me now list all four unhealthy beliefs before I discuss each in turn:

Unhealthy belief 1   Rigid demands
Unhealthy belief 2   Awfulizing
Unhealthy belief 3   Discomfort intolerance
Unhealthy belief 4   Depreciation

Unhealthy belief 1   Rigid demands

I have already discussed rigid demands, but as this issue is so important let me emphasize the points that I have already made. It is likely that you prefer certain conditions to exist before you begin work on a task. As we shall see, there is nothing wrong with having such preferences even if the conditions that you desire do not exist, for unmet preferences do not lead to procrastination. However, as humans we can easily transform our preferences into demands by insisting that the conditions we want to exist before beginning work on a task *absolutely must* exist. It is then that we are very likely to procrastinate because we are giving ourselves no room to manoeuvre at all. If we decree that a condition such as freedom from discomfort has to exist before we begin a task that it is in our best interests to do, then how are we to begin work on such a task if we do experience discomfort? The answer is that we are not. So as long as we hold rigid demands about conditions that have to exist before we get going, we will not get going if such conditions do not exist, and if they do exist we may still be vulnerable to procrastination because the situation may soon change and we may lose these conditions whose existence we deem so necessary for task performance. This is why Albert Ellis regards rigid demands as lying at the very core of procrastination.

Unhealthy belief 2   Awfulizing

When your rigid demands are not met, then you are likely to hold what we refer to in REBT as an awfulizing belief. When you hold such a belief you are making an extreme negative evaluation of the conditions that exist which you believe absolutely should not exist. Thus, if you believe that you must be comfortable before you begin to work on the task at hand, then if you do experience discomfort you will tend to believe that it is terrible to experience such discomfort, a belief that will lead you to get rid of the discomfort by procrastinating on the task at hand. Awfulizing beliefs often take the form of statements such as: 'It's awful that . . .', 'It's terrible that . . .' and 'It's the end of the world that . . .' The defining feature of an awfulizing belief is that at the time that you hold this belief, you really do believe that nothing can be worse.

Unhealthy belief 3   Discomfort intolerance

When your rigid demands are not met, you then tend to consider that you are unable to tolerate the ensuing situation. Thus, if you believe that you must not experience discomfort before starting the task at hand, and you begin to experience such discomfort, you will tend to think that you cannot put up with these uncomfortable feelings. Consequently, you will tend to put off doing the task in order to avoid experiencing discomfort.

Unhealthy belief 4   Depreciation

Depreciation beliefs can be held about the self, others or life conditions in general. When you hold a depreciation belief about yourself, you tend to put yourself down when you consider that you have acted in a way that you absolutely shouldn't or that you have not done what you believe you absolutely should have done. For example, a very common procrastination scenario occurs when you think about doing a task that you won't be able to do very well, and thus decide not to begin it or even think about beginning it. The reason why you procrastinate under these circumstances is that you believe that you have to do the task well and if you don't this will prove that you are a failure. The self-depreciating belief ('I am a failure') stems from your demand that you have to do the task well when you think that you will not be able to do so. Rather than think of yourself as a failure, you procrastinate instead.

When you hold a depreciation belief about another person, you consider that person to be bad or worthless, for example, either for doing something that you believe he absolutely should not have done or for not doing something that you believe he absolutely should have done. As I mentioned earlier, some people procrastinate to restore the balance between them and other people. For example, John was told to do something by his boss which was actually in his best interests to do, but John put off doing the task. He did so because he considered that his boss was wrong for ordering him to do the task, and rotten for doing so. Consequently, in order to get back at his boss (and thus restore a sense of balance in his mind) he put off starting on the task that his boss ordered him to do, even though doing so was against his own long-term best interests.

Finally, when you hold a depreciation belief about life conditions you are saying that conditions are rotten for being the way that they really must not be. The type of procrastination that stems from this depreciation belief is related to self-pity, where the person considers himself to be hard done by because life is giving him what he does not deserve (as it must not do) or is not giving him what he deserves (as it must do). Feeling sorry for himself because the world is a rotten uncaring place, the person seeks to cheer himself and is thus very unlikely to begin a task that is in any way onerous. Rather, he will turn to activities that are enjoyable in the short term.

Having discussed the four unhealthy beliefs that underpin the different types of procrastination, I will now go on to discuss the four healthy alternatives to these beliefs.

The four healthy alternative beliefs that will help you to overcome chronic procrastination

So far I have discussed the four unhealthy beliefs that lead to both types of chronic procrastination (specific and general). In this section, I will discuss healthy alternatives to these four beliefs that will help you to overcome your chronic procrastination problem. These four healthy beliefs are as follows:

Healthy belief 1   Full preferences
Healthy belief 2   Anti-awfulizing
Healthy belief 3   Discomfort tolerance
Healthy belief 4   Acceptance

There are three reasons that these beliefs are healthy. First, they are consistent with reality (i.e. they are true); second, they make sense; and third, they are helpful (in this context they lead to task execution rather than to procrastination). I will now discuss each of these healthy beliefs in turn.

Healthy belief 1   Full preferences

As I mentioned earlier, it is healthy for humans to have preferences. However, if we take a closer look at the concept of a preference we have to distinguish between partial preferences and full preferences. Partial preferences outline what a person wants to happen (e.g. 'I want to do well') or wants not to happen (e.g. 'I don't want to experience discomfort') and that is all. Full preferences, on the other hand, not only outline what a person wants to happen, but acknowledge that there is no reason why that desire has to be met (e.g. 'I want to do well, but I don't have to do so'). Additionally, full preferences not only outline what the person prefers not to happen, they also indicate that there is no reason why this must not occur (e.g. 'I don't want to experience discomfort, but there is no reason why I have to be free of this experience'). Whereas rigid demands give you no leeway in a task-related situation (e.g. 'I absolutely must be free from discomfort before I start working on my tax return forms') and thereby often lead to procrastination, full preferences are flexible and allow you to proceed even if your immediate preferences are not met ('I want to be free from discomfort before I start working on my tax return forms, but it is not necessary for me to be comfortable prior to getting down to this onerous task').

Healthy belief 2   Anti-awfulizing

When your full preferences are not met, then you are likely to hold what we refer to in REBT as an anti-awfulizing belief. When you hold such a belief you are making a non-extreme negative evaluation of the undesirable conditions that exist, but you do not demand that they absolutely should not exist. Thus, if you believe that it would be preferable, but not necessary, for you to be comfortable before you begin to work on the task at hand, then if you do experience discomfort you will tend to believe that it is bad, but not terrible, to experience such discomfort, a belief that will lead you to getting down to do the task. Anti-awfulizing beliefs often take the form of statements such as 'It's bad, but not awful that . . .', 'It's unfortunate, but not terrible that . . .' and 'It's crummy, but not the end of the world that . . .' The defining feature of anti-awfulizing belief is summed up by what Smokey Robinson's mother used to tell her son: 'From the day you were born, 'til you ride in the hearse, there's nothing so bad that it couldn't be worse.'

Healthy belief 3   Discomfort tolerance

When your full preferences are not met, you then tend to consider that you are able to tolerate the ensuing situation even though it may be difficult for you to do so. Thus, if you believe that you'd rather not experience discomfort before starting the task at hand, but that there is no law decreeing that you must be free from discomfort before you start, and you begin to experience such discomfort, you will tend to think that you can put up with these uncomfortable feelings, even though it is tough to do so. Critically, you will then remind yourself that it is, in fact, in your interests for you to tolerate your discomfort. If you do this you will begin the task even though you are uncomfortable. Discomfort tolerance beliefs, therefore, will aid you in your attempt to overcome your chronic procrastination.

33

Healthy belief 4   Acceptance

Acceptance beliefs, like depreciation beliefs, can be held about the self, others or life conditions in general. When you hold an acceptance belief about yourself, you accept yourself as an unrateable, fallible human being for acting in a way that you deem undesirable, but not absolutely forbidden, or for not doing something that you would have preferred rather than insisted to have done. For example, when you think about doing a task and think that you may not be able to do it, when you accept yourself for possibly not being able to do it, you will still attempt it because it is in your interests to do so. Your self-accepting belief ('I am a fallible human being even if I fail at the task') stems from your full preference that you want to do the task well, but don't have to do so. This leads you to begin the task rather than procrastinate.

When you hold an acceptance belief about another person, you consider that person to be an unrateable, fallible human being for either doing something that you believe he preferably should not have done or for not doing something that you believe he preferably should have done. When John was told to do something by his boss which was actually in his best interests to do, he did it even though he considered that his boss was wrong for ordering him to do the task. He did so because he considered his boss to be a fallible human being who did the wrong thing rather than a bad person for doing so. Thus, an other-acceptance belief helps you to overcome chronic procrastination.

Finally, when you hold an acceptance about life conditions you are saying that conditions are a mixture of good, bad and neutral aspects even though you prefer (but do not demand) that they be different. Thus, when a person considers that life is giving him what he does not deserve (which he prefers, but does not insist, that it not do) or is not giving him what he deserves (as again he prefers, but does not demand, that it do), he is disappointed, but not disturbed, about this grim reality. Believing this, the person will do the task in question when it is in his best interests to do so even if he finds it onerous. Having done so, he will then turn to activities that are enjoyable, which is a major feature of an anti-procrastination strategy.

5
Developing an Anti-procrastination Strategy

I have devoted quite a lot of space to discussing the point that you procrastinate not because of the conditions that you face (or anticipate facing), but largely because of the beliefs that you hold about these conditions. I then went on to outline the four unhealthy beliefs that lie at the core of chronic procrastination, and the four healthy alternatives to these unhealthy beliefs. These healthy beliefs are the cornerstone of what may be called an anti-procrastination philosophy. But how do you acquire such a philosophy? It would be nice if your brain was like a computer so that you could remove the chronic procrastination program (comprised of the four unhealthy beliefs) and replace it with the anti-procrastination program (containing the four healthy beliefs), but the human brain does not work like that. How, then, can you change your unhealthy beliefs? You do so by questioning both your unhealthy and your healthy beliefs and by seeing which stand the test of such scrutiny. Then you strengthen your healthy beliefs, and finally you act on them. Let me start by showing you how to question your beliefs.

Question your beliefs

Here you take the following three steps.

Step 1   Identify your unhealthy beliefs

In order to identify the unhealthy beliefs that underpin your procrastination, whenever you put off doing something that is in your best interests to do, ask yourself the following questions while keenly imagining a specific episode of your chronic procrastination.

1 What conditions am I insisting have to exist before I begin work on the task?
2 Am I telling myself that it would be awful if these conditions did not exist?
3 Can I bear it if these conditions do not exist?
4 Is depreciating myself, others or life conditions a central feature of my procrastination?

If you identify one or more unhealthy beliefs, write them down and put them in your own words.

Step 2   Write down the healthy alternatives to your unhealthy beliefs

Once you have written down your unhealthy beliefs, write down the healthy alternative next to each unhealthy belief. Here are some examples:

- *Unhealthy belief (rigid demand)*: I must know that my father will approve of the work I do on the task before I start to work on it.
- *Healthy belief (full preference)*: I'd like to know that my father will approve of the work I do on the task, *but* I don't need to know this before I begin to work on the task.

- *Unhealthy belief (awfulizing belief)*: It's terrible to be told to do something by my boss without being consulted.
- *Healthy belief (anti-awfulizing belief)*: It's bad to be told to do something by my boss without being consulted, *but* it is not terrible.

- *Unhealthy belief (discomfort intolerance)*: I can't stand to experience the discomfort of doing something onerous even if it is worth doing.
- *Healthy belief (discomfort tolerance)*: It is difficult putting up with the discomfort of doing something onerous that is worth doing, *but* I can stand it and it is worth tolerating.

- *Unhealthy belief (self-depreciation belief)*: If I fail to get a good grade on my essay, it proves that I am a failure.
- *Healthy belief (self-acceptance belief)*: If I fail to get a good grade on my essay, it does not prove that I am a failure. Not getting a good grade does not diminish my worth as a person. I am the same fallible, unrateable person whether I get a good grade or not.

- *Unhealthy belief (other-depreciation belief)*: My supervisor is a rotten person for asking me to make the changes to my thesis when I think my work is OK.
- *Healthy belief (other-acceptance belief)*: My supervisor is not a rotten person for asking me to make the changes to my thesis when I think my work is OK. He is a fallible human being who I think is mistaken in his views.

- *Unhealthy belief (depreciating life conditions)*: Life stinks for giving me so much work to do.

• *Healthy belief (accepting life conditions)*: Life does not stink for giving me so much work to do. Life is complex, made up of good things, bad things and neutral things.

Step 3   Question your unhealthy and healthy beliefs

This next step is really important and lies at the heart of overcoming chronic procrastination. It involves subjecting both your unhealthy and your healthy beliefs to scrutiny on three issues: the empirical issue (i.e. whether a belief is true or false); the logical issue (i.e. whether a belief makes sense or not) and the pragmatic issue (i.e. whether the consequences of holding a belief are constructive or unconstructive). Let me give you two examples of how this is done.

Questioning rigid demands and full preferences

• *Rigid demand*: I must know that my father will approve of the work I do on the task before I start to work on it.

• *Full preference*: I'd like to know that my father will approve of the work I do on the task, but I don't need to know this before I begin to work on the task.

Question 1 (empirical issue): Which belief is true and which is false? *Answer*: My rigid demand is false and my full preference is true. If my demand were true, this would mean that I could not possibly start work on the task until I knew that my father approved of what I did on the task. However, as it is possible for me to begin the task without knowing this, my demand is not consistent with reality.

My full preference, on the other hand, is true. I really would like to know that my father would approve of my task performance before I started work on it, so that is true. It is also true that there is no law of the universe decreeing that I have to know this.

Question 2 (logical issue): Which belief is logical/sensible and which is not? *Answer*: My rigid demand is not logical whereas my full preference makes sense. If we start with my full preference, this contains two parts, one which states what I want: 'I'd like to know that my father will approve of the work I do on the task' (known as the partial preference); and one which negates my demand: '. . . but I don't have to know this before I begin to work on the task'. Both parts of my full

37

preference are flexible and therefore logically connected together. However, my rigid demand does not follow logically from my partial preference: 'I'd like to know that my father will approve of the work I do on the task . . . and therefore I have to know' and it certainly doesn't follow logically from my full preference: 'I'd like to know that my father will approve of the work I do on the task, but I don't need to know this before I begin to work on the task . . . and therefore I must know that my father will approve of the work I do on the task before I start to work on it.' You cannot logically derive a rigid statement from a flexible statement.

Question 3 (pragmatic issue): Which belief is helpful to me (in this context, helps me to get started on the task) and which is not helpful to me (in this context, leads to procrastination)?
Answer: My rigid demand is not helpful to me whereas my full preference will help me. If I believe that I have to know that my father will approve of what I do before I do it, the only way I can start the task is to know in advance how well I am going to perform the task and what my father's response will be to my task performance. Since I cannot know either of these things in advance I will not be able to begin working at the task as long as I hold this belief. Thus, my rigid demand will lead me to procrastinate. However, if I stop demanding that I have to know that my father will approve of me before I begin the task, but keep this as a full preference, then this desire only stipulates what conditions I would prefer to exist before I start the task, not the conditions that have to exist before I get going. Thus, when I am faced with undesirable conditions (in this case not knowing whether or not my father will approve of me), my full preference gives me the flexibility to start the task under these conditions, whereas my rigid demand does not give me such flexibility. Thus, my full preference helps me to begin the task, especially if I deem that it is in my best interests to do so.

Strengthen your healthy beliefs

Once you have gained practice at questioning the unhealthy beliefs that underpin your chronic procrastination and the healthy alternative beliefs that will help you to get going, you can probably understand that your unhealthy beliefs are false, illogical and unhelpful to you and that your alternative healthy beliefs are true, logical and helpful. However, your understanding of these points is likely only to be intellectual in nature. People who only have intellectual understanding of these issues typically say that they understand these points in their heads, but they don't really believe them in their hearts. Such intellectual understanding, while an important first step in overcoming chronic procrastination, does not usually lead to a change in feeling or behaviour. The type of understanding that does lead to a change in feeling and behaviour is called emotional understanding and is reflected in statements such as: 'I really understand that I don't need to know that my father will approve of me for my task performance before I begin to work on the task, and thus I am going to begin the task because doing so is in my best interests.' In this statement, the person demonstrates a deep conviction in the healthy belief and can act on it.

In this section, I will describe two techniques for facilitating emotional understanding of healthy beliefs, and in the following section I will discuss the importance of acting in a way that is consistent with these new beliefs.

The attack–response technique

One powerful way of strengthening your healthy beliefs is to attack them and respond effectively to these attacks. This technique is called the attack–response technique, and here is a set of instructions for how to use it.

1 Write down the healthy belief that you wish to strengthen on a piece of paper.
2 Rate your present level of conviction in this healthy belief on a 100-point scale with 0 per cent = no conviction and 100 per cent = total conviction, and write down this rating below the belief.
3 Attack this healthy belief as genuinely as you can. This attack will probably take the form of another unhealthy belief or a doubt, reservation or objection to the healthy belief. Write down this attack below the conviction rating.
4 Respond to this attack as fully as you can. It is really important that you respond to each element of this attack. Do so as persuasively as possible and write down this response below this attack.
5 Continue in this vein until you have answered all your attacks and cannot think of any more.

If you find this exercise difficult, you might find it easier to make your attacks gently at first. Then, when you find that you can respond to these attacks quite easily, begin to make the attacks more biting. Work in this way until you are making really strong attacks. When you make an attack, do so as if you want yourself to believe it. Similarly, when you respond to your attacks, really throw yourself into it with the intention of demolishing the attack and raising your level of conviction in your healthy belief.

Don't forget that the purpose of the exercise is to strengthen your healthy belief, so it is important that you stop when you have answered all of your attacks.

6 When you have answered all of your attacks, write down your original healthy belief (i.e. the belief you want to strengthen) and then re-rate your level of conviction in it using the same 100-point scale that you employed before. You will probably find that this rating has gone up. If it hasn't, look again at what you wrote and see if you can spot occasions when you didn't respond to an attack or an element of the attack, or spot instances where your responses to attacks were not persuasive. In either case, re-do that part of the attack–response sequence until your new conviction rating has increased.

Let me demonstrate how one person used this technique to good effect. Bernard suffered from chronic procrastination in the area of keeping his files up to date. He understood clearly that it was in his best interests to do so and also acknowledged that despite seeing this he continued to procrastinate in this area because he held the following unhealthy belief: 'I have to be in the right frame of mind before I do my filing.' Bernard followed the steps that I outlined in the previous section. After identifying this unhealthy belief, he formulated the following alternative healthy belief: 'I would prefer to be in the right frame of mind before I did my filing, but it isn't necessary for me to do so. I can begin filing even though I don't "feel like" doing it, and it is in my best interests to do just that.' Bernard then questioned both these beliefs and began to understand that his unhealthy belief was false, illogical and unhelpful to him in the sense that it led to procrastination, and that his alternative rational belief was, by contrast, consistent with reality, sensible and helpful in the sense that it would promote constructive action. However, he still continued to procrastinate because he said that while he could understand why healthy belief was healthy, he didn't really believe it yet. It was at this point that I taught him how to use the attack–response technique and this is what he did.

Healthy belief: 'I would prefer to be in the right frame of mind before I did my filing, but it isn't necessary for me to do so. I can begin filing even though I don't "feel like" doing it and it is in my best interests to do just that.'
Conviction rating: 40 per cent.

Attack: Come off it. If I do it when I am not in the right frame of mind, it's terrible. Better to wait until I want to do it.
Response: Let's face it, doing filing when I am not up for it is pretty bad, but that hardly means it is terrible. I can think of many things that are worse, and terrible means nothing can be worse. That's ludicrous. Also, if I wait until I want to do the filing I'll wait for a very long time, and if I do this, the filing will build up and the chances that I will want to do filing when the pile is huge are far less than when the pile is small.

Attack: Yes, but doing filing is uncomfortable and I can't bear this discomfort.
Response: I agree that it is uncomfortable doing filing because it is hardly a pleasurable task, but that doesn't mean that I can't bear it. Of course I can bear it, it's hardly going to kill me.

Attack: Yes, but filing is such a menial task, I shouldn't have to do it.
Response: OK, so filing is a menial task, but that doesn't mean that I can be spared doing it. I am not so grand that I should be exempt from filing. Also, if I do menial tasks this doesn't make me a menial, lowly person. I'm the same person whether I do the filing or not, and it clearly is in my best interests to do it and to do it regularly so I am on top of my business affairs.

Attack: But it's so unfair. I work hard at my business. I shouldn't have to put up with the unfairness of filing.
Response: First, doing filing is part of my business. Just because I do some of my business tasks well doesn't mean that it is unfair that I have to do my own filing. But even if it is unfair, who says that I have to be spared unfairness? I don't have to be thus spared. However, if I demand that I do have to be spared I will have three problems for the price of one: the filing, my disturbance about the unfairness of doing it, and the procrastination which will result from my disturbance.

Original healthy belief: 'I would prefer to be in the right frame of mind before I did my filing, but it isn't necessary for me to do so. I can begin filing even though I don't "feel like" doing it and it is in my best interests to do just that.'
Conviction re-rating: 75 per cent.

There are two other variations of the attack–response technique that you might wish to use. The first involves you putting your attacks and responses on to an audiotape so that when you replay the dialogue you can evaluate not only the content of the arguments that you employed, but the tone in which you made them. It is important that the tone of your responses is more powerful and convincing than the tone of your attacks. If the reverse is the case then your conviction ratings in your healthy belief will not go up and may even go down. Thus, when you are using the tape-recorded version of the attack–response technique, try to make your responses sound more powerful and persuasive than your attacks, by modifying your tone of voice accordingly.

The second variation of the attack–response technique that I want to mention is known as the devil's advocate technique. This technique involves you enlisting the help of a friend. Ask your friend to attack your healthy belief in the way that you did in the written and tape-recorded versions of the technique, while your task is to respond to their attacks. You may have to explain the nature of healthy and unhealthy beliefs to your friend before they are able to play the role of devil's advocate properly, but if done well this technique can help you to strengthen your healthy beliefs in a powerful way.

I am often asked whether the three variations of the attack–response technique should be done in any set order. While there is no absolute set order, I do recommend that you do the written variation first, followed by the tape-recorded variation, while the devil's advocate variation should be used last. I recommend this order because in my experience it best facilitates competency in the use of the attack–response technique. However, if you find that a different order works better for you, then by all means use your own judgement.

The emotive-imagery technique

A second method of strengthening your healthy belief is known as the emotive-imagery technique. Here are the instructions that I usually give people who wish to strengthen their anti-procrastination healthy belief.

1 Identify a situation where you procrastinated and identify the theme of your procrastination (see pp. 21–25 for a discussion of procrastination themes). This may have been a threat (such as discomfort, the prospect of failure or disapproval), a state of imbalance with another person, or lack of motivation (i.e. procrastination as prelude), to name but three.

2 Close your eyes and vividly imagine this situation and focus on the theme of your procrastination.

3 Identify and get in touch with the unhealthy belief that you held about this theme.

4 While still imagining the same situation and focusing on the same theme, change your unhealthy belief to its healthy alternative and stay with this new belief until you see yourself beginning the task that you procrastinated on.

5 Keep this healthy belief and associated action in your mind's eye for about five minutes, all the time imagining the theme that you have identified. If you go back to the former unhealthy belief, bring the new one back.

In using the emotive-imagery technique, Bernard closed his eyes and imagined facing a pile of filing that it was in his interests to do. In doing so, he focused on the uncomfortable aspects of approaching the task (since 'discomfort' was the theme of Bernard's procrastination) and got in touch with both his unhealthy belief ('I have to be in the right frame of mind before I do my filing') and the strong tendency to procrastinate that went hand-in-hand with his belief. Then, while keeping his focus on the discomfort that he associated with the pile of filing in front of him, again in his mind's eye, Bernard changed to his alternative healthy belief ('I would prefer to be in the right frame of mind before I did my filing, but it isn't necessary for me to do so. I can begin filing even though I don't "feel like" doing it and it is in my best interests to do just that') and maintained that belief for five minutes while at the same time picturing himself doing his filing.

Since this technique only takes about seven minutes to do, I suggest that you practise it several times a day. You can do it while waiting for a bus or as you travel to and from work on the train. As you develop competence in this, I suggest that you do it about ten times a day, especially if you experience chronic general procrastination, until you are able to stop procrastinating in practice. However, please do not use this technique in the service of your procrastination (i.e. don't practise the technique instead of doing the task – practise it as a prelude to taking action).

Act on your healthy beliefs

In the previous section, I described two major ways of strengthening your healthy beliefs: the attack–response technique and the emotive-imagery technique. Both of these techniques are cognitive techniques in that when using them you are employing your thinking capacity and your imagination. However, unless you act on these beliefs you will not incorporate your healthy beliefs into your belief system and you will continue to procrastinate. Thus, after you have strengthened your beliefs cognitively, it is important that you do so behaviourally. In doing so, I suggest that you rehearse your new healthy beliefs at the same time as you take action, while confronting the situation and the theme that you usually respond to with procrastination.

For example, after Bernard (who I first discussed in the previous section) strengthened his healthy belief by using the attack–response technique and the emotive-imagery technique, he strengthened it behaviourally, by beginning to do his filing when he was not in the right frame of mind to do so, while rehearsing his healthy belief (i.e. 'I would prefer to be in the right frame of mind before I did my filing, but it isn't necessary for me to do so. I can begin filing even though I don't "feel like" doing it and it is in my best interests to do just that').

If Bernard had strengthened his healthy belief cognitively, but whenever he didn't 'feel like' filing he did not act on this belief, then he would have ended up by weakening this belief and strengthening his unhealthy belief (i.e. 'I have to be in the right frame of mind before I do my filing'). In this case, even though Bernard would have been rehearsing his healthy belief cognitively, his failure to do his filing when he was not in the frame of mind to do so would have proved to him, albeit erroneously, that he really does need to feel in the right frame of mind before he begins to do his filing.

Thus, I strongly suggest that after you have strengthened your healthy belief cognitively, you act on your healthy, anti-procrastination belief and do so without delay. For if you delay, you will tend to strengthen your old procrastination-based unhealthy belief, which is, of course, the last thing that you want to do. The more you respond with immediate action to instances where you would have procrastinated in the past (while rehearsing your healthy belief at the same time), the more likely it is that you will overcome your chronic procrastination. The more you delay, however, in such instances, the more likely it is that you will undermine all the work that you have done to change your healthy beliefs to date, with the consequence that you will continue to put off until tomorrow tasks that it is in your best interests to do today.

In this part of the book I have discussed how to deal with chronic procrastination in general terms. In the next part I will cover specific types of chronic procrastination. In doing so, I will discuss the psychological factors that are common in each of the specific types, and how to deal with them. As these are variations on what I have discussed in the first part of the book, I suggest that you re-read relevant sections as you proceed.

PART 2

Dealing with Different Types
of Procrastination

6

Dealing with 'Just So' Procrastination

As I mentioned above, in this part of the book I will discuss how you can deal with different types of procrastination. In doing so, the techniques that I suggest should be viewed as complementing the techniques that I taught you in the first part.

If you experience chronic 'just so' procrastination, it is very likely that you put things off because you fear that if you did them they would not be 'just so'. People who experience this type of procrastination tend to think of themselves as perfectionistic, and while they can see the dangers of procrastination, they may well have mixed feelings about giving up their perfectionistic ideas, believing erroneously that this means that they will have to settle for second best.

How can you judge whether you suffer from 'just so' procrastination? You do so if you exhibit most of the following characteristics either some or most of the time.

1 You tend to think in black-and-white terms (e.g. 'either what I do is perfect or it is rubbish').
2 You won't begin doing something until all the conditions are 'just so'.
3 You are highly competitive and believe that you have to be number one, and unless you are sure of doing so, you won't begin doing the task at hand.
4 You believe that there is a right way and a wrong way of doing something, and unless you are sure that you will do something the right way then you won't do it at all, even though doing it is in your best interests.
5 You believe that excellence (which you demand you have to achieve) has to be achieved without too much effort, and if you have to struggle at something it means that you are no good at it.
6 You believe that your performances and your abilities determine your self-worth.
7 You think that you have to do the task in one go and if you think that you can't then you won't do it at all.
8 Once you have started a task, in your quest to do it perfectly well, you spend far more time on the task than it warrants. Before

49

you begin a task, knowing how much time you tend to spend on such tasks discourages you from beginning the task in question.

9 Once you begin a task, you tend to monitor your task performance very closely, and if what you have just done is not 'just so', you will go back and do it again. In this way you tend to make very slow progress once you have begun a task.

10 You tend not to ask for help if things go wrong, believing that this will reveal you to be a weak person. In addition, from your perfectionistic frame of reference you consider that when others help you, what you do doesn't count.

So far I have discussed the perfectionistic type of 'just so' procrastination. There is another type of 'just so' procrastination which reflects an obsessive-compulsive type of procrastination. If you experience this type of procrastination:

1 You will not do anything if it means that you are not in full control either of yourself or of the conditions under which you are working. In taking this stance, you tend to think that you will lose complete control of yourself if you slacken the tight reins of total self-control, and that if you fail to control your environment, chaos will ensue.

2 You will not do the task unless you are absolutely sure of how it will turn out.

3 You regard yourself as fully responsible for the outcome of your performance and you won't do the task in case it turns out badly. If it does, you will blame yourself for producing the bad outcome.

4 You refuse to take risks and will put off doing the task until there is no risk involved in doing so.

5 You refuse to delegate tasks to others because you don't trust them to do it 'just so'. Thus, you are often overwhelmed with tasks that you insist only you are allowed to carry out. This means that you rarely get to tasks that are important for you to do on time. Consequently, you constantly have the sense that you are chasing your own tail.

In order to tackle perfectionistic 'just so' procrastination, it is important that you do the following:

● Stop thinking in black-and-white terms and start practising viewing events as existing along a continuum. For example, instead of thinking 'either what I do is perfect or it is rubbish', show yourself that there are many points between 'perfect' and 'rubbish'.

- Challenge the idea that all the conditions have to be 'just so' before you begin doing something that is in your best interests to do and practise acting in a way that is inconsistent with this idea.
- Challenge the idea that you have to be the best at doing something and show yourself that you can do a task even though others may do better at it than you.
- Realize that in many cases there are several ways of doing something and that there is not a right way and a wrong way of doing it.
- Appreciate that excellence is often achieved after much dedicated striving and is rarely reached effortlessly.
- Develop a philosophy of self-acceptance in which your self-worth is based on you being human, alive and unique rather than on your excellent performances and your abilities.
- Appreciate that while you may do something perfectly well, you will only be able to do so once in a while. Torvill and Dean may have been able to achieve a perfect 6.0 at ice dancing, but if they had had to perform the same dance immediately after their perfect performance, they would not have done as well, because they would have been drained from their previous efforts.
- Acknowledge that it is in the nature of being human to make mistakes and that you don't have to give up on something once you have made an error. Rather, you can learn from your errors and continue doing the task in question.
- Before you begin the task and as you do it, focus on what is realistic rather than on what is ideal.
- Don't give up your high standards, but do give up your demand that you always have to achieve these standards.
- Give up the demand that you have to do the task in one go. Many tasks, unless they are simple and routine, often take more than one 'sitting' to be completed. If you accept this and are prepared to leave a task unfinished for a while, then this will help you to overcome your procrastination.
- If you are perfectionistic in your thinking, it is particularly important for you to set a realistic time limit to complete the task. Otherwise you will spend too much time on the task, once you have started it, and this will help to reinforce your perfectionism since the main reason you are allotting so much time to the task is that you are trying to do it perfectly well.
- Once you have begun a task, it is very important that you don't review it until you have finished it. In this way you will tend to

undercut your habit of going over old ground several times in an attempt to do everything that you do 'just so'.

● Dispute the idea that asking for help means that you are a weak person. Rather, show yourself that it means that you are a fallible human being with strengths and weaknesses and occasionally you need others to help you to do something. Remember this phrase: 'Only you can do it, but you don't have to do it alone.' Thinking this way will make complex tasks less daunting, and thus you are more likely to tackle them if you know that you can call on others for help.

In tackling obsessive-compulsive based procrastination, you will want to make use of several of the strategies that I have referred to when discussing tackling perfectionistic procrastination. In addition, I suggest that you do the following:

1 Get used to tolerating not being totally in control, either of yourself or of the conditions under which you are working. Begin the task anyway. You will soon learn that you will not fall apart if you do this on a regular basis, nor will chaos inevitably follow occasions when you let go of controlling your environment.

2 Challenge the idea that you need to know how something will turn out before you do it. Recognize that having such knowledge is fine, but you don't need it, which is good because you will rarely if ever have such foresight. If we did, bookmakers would not exist because we would be betting on certainties. Get used to dealing with probabilities rather than guarantees. It's uncomfortable doing so, but it is tolerable and such discomfort is well worth putting up with because it will help you to overcome your chronic procrastination.

3 Recognize that if you do something wrong, it is important to take responsibility for your actions, but without blaming yourself for them. If you have particular difficulty in this area, I suggest that you consult my book entitled *Overcoming Guilt* (Sheldon Press, 1994). In that book I describe in detail how responsibility plus blame leads you to take an excessive amount of responsibility for the outcomes of your actions, whereas responsibility plus self-acceptance leads you to take an appropriate amount of responsibility for them and give others involved some responsibility too. The latter philosophy will help you to overcome your chronic responsibility where obsessive-compulsiveness and guilt are involved.

4 Gradually get used to taking risks while tolerating the great

discomfort you are likely to experience as you do so. Starting something may well seem like a big risk to you, but if you do so you will begin to get used to taking risks, especially if you take the horror out of anything that goes wrong – as it will from time to time, because that, unfortunately from your point of view, is life.

5 Begin to delegate tasks to others and trust them to do their best. This may well not be 'the best', or 'your best', but it will often do, especially in the long term. I know you cringe when you think about tolerating less than the best from yourself and from others, but if you take the awfulness out of this situation you will see that it will help you to overcome your procrastination problem.

To reiterate, delegating tasks to others will ultimately lighten your load in the longer term, particularly if you are prepared to accept good to excellent work from people rather than only perfection. If you delegate while changing your own attitude towards perfection in yourself and in others, then you are more likely to do things on time, because you will have less to do in your life.

7

Dealing with Procrastination Based on Fear of Failure

If you experience chronic procrastination based on fear of failure, you put things off when you think that you might fail at something. The difference between this type of procrastination and perfectionistic procrastination is that in the latter you are anxious about doing things imperfectly, whereas in the former you are anxious about failing. There are similarities between the two, because in perfectionistic procrastination you often think that less than perfect performance is equivalent to failure.

How can you judge if you suffer from procrastination based on fear of failure? You do so if you exhibit most of the following characteristics either some or most of the time.

- You hold the rigid demand that you must not fail or do poorly at the task in question.
- You tend to equate your worth in terms of your performance. Thus, if you fail or do poorly at something important to you, then you will think of yourself as a failure.
- When you think of doing the task in question you overestimate the odds that you will fail at the task or do it poorly.
- You won't begin doing something until you are sure that you won't fail at it.
- Once you begin a task, you tend to monitor your task performance very closely. If you begin to struggle at it, you quickly conclude that this means that you will fail and thus you stop working at the task at hand.

In order to tackle procrastination based on fear of failure, it is important that you do the following:

1 Challenge and keep challenging your rigid demand that you must not fail or do poorly at the tasks that are in your best interests to do, and develop and strengthen the healthy alternative to this belief – that it is better to succeed than to fail, but there is no law exempting you

54

from failing. Given this, show yourself that it is better to risk failure than to guarantee it by not doing the task at all and, above all, act on these principles.

2 Show yourself repeatedly that your worth is not defined by your performance. Thus, if you do fail or do poorly at the task at hand, remind yourself that it is unfortunate that you did so, but this does not, repeat does not, mean that you are a failure. Rather, it means that you are a fallible human being who is capable of succeeding as well as failing. Again, it is important that you act on this principle and do so consistently.

3 Get the odds of failure and success into proportion. Is it really a dead cert that you are going to fail? If a good friend of yours had the same ability at the task as you, would you advise her not to do the task because she was bound to fail? If not, why not base the odds of your success and failure on the same sober analysis and then begin doing the task at hand?

4 Challenge the idea that you have to be sure of success before you start. There is no such certainty, and demanding it will only have one result – procrastination. We only have probability, and it is important that you accept this and act accordingly.

5 Once you begin a task, learn to concentrate on what you are doing rather than on how you are doing. The former will help you to keep working at the task in question, whereas the latter will reinforce your fear of failure and increase the chances that you will stop soon after you have started.

8

Dealing with Procrastination Based on 'Fear of Success'

Strange as it seems at first glance, some people procrastinate not because they fear failure, but because they fear success. Rather than doing something and risking succeeding or doing well on the task, if you fear success you will find ways of putting off doing whatever it is that it is in your interests to do.

Actually, fear of success as a concept doesn't really capture what the person is afraid of, in the same way that fear of flying doesn't capture what people are afraid of when they take an aeroplane flight. In the latter case, they may be afraid of the plane crashing or of being shut in a confined space with no ready means of escape, but they are not afraid that the plane is going to fly. In the same way, if you fear success you are not afraid that you are going to succeed at something; rather, you are afraid of the implications of success or of what might happen after you have done well at the task at hand.

Let me now take a closer look at what you might really be afraid of if you succeed at something, and how you can deal with this fear if it applies to you.

First, you may be afraid that if you succeed at something then significant others will expect a lot more of you, and you believe under such circumstances that you have to live up to their expectations. If you hold such a belief, you will reason with yourself that it is better to procrastinate and thus not risk success than to do the task, perform well at it and later fail to live up to others' expectations. The main way of dealing with this fear is to challenge the belief that you have to live up to the expectations of significant others. Wanting to live up to the expectations of others is fine as long as you remind yourself that it isn't essential to do so. Holding this full preference won't stop you from doing the task in the first place, while believing that you have to meet the expectations of others will. I will have more to say on this issue in the next chapter when I deal with approval-based procrastination.

Second, you may fear that if you do a task and are successful at it then you will outdo someone you care for. You think that in such cases they will be upset and you will be to blame. Believing this, you privately reason that it is better to procrastinate than to do the task, perform it well and then be responsible for another's hurt. This belief is common in those who experience much guilt in their lives. Such people take far too much responsibility for events in their lives and give others who are involved far too little responsibility. The way to deal with this fear is to assume initially that your success will lead to another's distress and that you are partly responsible for this, and then challenge the idea that your behaviour must never result in the distress of others. Second, you need to challenge the idea that you are a bad person if you are responsible for the distress of another. That would be a bad thing to have done, but are you really a bad person for doing so? Of course not. You are fallible and sometimes you will hurt someone's feelings. Having disputed your rigid demand and self-depreciation belief, you are now in a position to look at the issue of responsibility more objectively. If you do well and another person is upset by it, what are you responsible for and what is the other person responsible for? My argument is that you are responsible for your behaviour and the other person is responsible for their response to your success. When you feel guilty about another's response to your success, you take responsibility for both your behaviour and the other person's response. If this were so, then if they did well and you were upset they would be responsible for your feelings. I hope you can see that this isn't the case. And if it isn't the case you cannot be responsible for the other person's feelings about your success. By all means be concerned about the feelings of others, but don't sacrifice yourself to spare the other person's feelings. Otherwise you will continue procrastinating for a long time to come. If you think that guilt plays a large role in your chronic procrastination, you might find it useful to read my book *Overcoming Guilt* (Sheldon Press, 1994).

Third, you may fear that if you do the task in question and do well at it then you may be hurt yourself. For example, Naomi feared that if she studied and did well at her exams then her friends, who all avoided studying like the plague, would boycott her or be nasty to her. I helped Naomi over her procrastination problem by encouraging her to see that if her friends did in fact respond in the way she predicted if she studied and did well in her exams, then this was unfortunate but hardly the end of the world. I then helped Naomi to acknowledge that she did have career aspirations that were important to her and if her friends did not support her in her plans then perhaps they were not true friends. So if you procrastinate because you fear that you may be hurt in some way as a result of succeeding at tasks, then take the horror out of these consequences and act in your best interests by doing as well as you can at the task in question.

Finally, you may fear success because you may think that you do not deserve to succeed or that you are not meant to succeed. The first of these reasons is based on the pernicious idea that your worth is based on something and if you do not achieve this something, then you do not deserve other advantages like success. If you believe this then it is important that you challenge it vigorously and often. As I pointed out earlier in the book, if you have worth as a human being then the only rational approach to human worth is to base your worth on aspects about you that don't change, like your humanness, aliveness and uniqueness. If you do this then you will overcome this fear, because the only way you stop deserving to succeed is to stop being human and unique or to die. However, if you base your deservingness on aspects that do change (e.g. pleasing your parents) then your deserving success is going to depend on your prior achievement of these conditions (i.e. you deserve success if you please your parents and you don't deserve success if you fail to please them). This is hardly a healthy way to live your life, and it certainly won't help you to overcome your procrastination problem in a sustained manner.

When you believe that you are not meant to succeed, you are frequently keeping alive a childhood message. Either you have accepted this idea from significant people in your childhood, or you are keeping alive a family rule (e.g. 'We Baxters aren't meant to succeed. I'm a Baxter, therefore I don't deserve to succeed'). In either case it is important to think critically about this idea. Ask yourself why you are not meant to succeed. If the answer is because your parents always said that you would be a failure, challenge this idea. Show yourself that your parents were wrong about this if this was their view. You have a perfect 'right' to succeed because you are human, and you don't have to keep alive the critical, biased and poisonous messages from your parents. Take responsibility for keeping this idea alive for yourself and learn to challenge it vigorously and often. If you think that you are not meant to succeed because you are a member of a family who are not meant to succeed, realize that you are not bound by this rule. Such family rules can be broken. Why can't you be the first Baxter to succeed? Why can't you re-write the old Baxter family rule? If you do, you will not only be helping yourself, you will be helping future generations of Baxters.

Before I conclude this chapter, let me stress a point that I have made before and will continue to repeat again and again. The only way to really change unhealthy beliefs is to act against them, and the only way to really internalize healthy beliefs is to act in ways that are consistent with them.

9

Dealing with Approval-based Procrastination

When you consistently put things off, it may be because you fear that should you do a particular task, then in some way you will incur the disapproval of people whom you deem to be important to you. It may seem that you are afraid to fail (see above), but the only reason you are scared of failure is because of the disapproval you are pretty sure you will face.

How can you judge whether you suffer from 'approval-based' procrastination? You do so if you exhibit most of the following characteristics either some or most of the time.

1 You believe that you must have the approval of people whom you deem to be significant to you. A related (but not identical) belief is when you demand that you must not incur the disapproval of significant people. The difference between these beliefs lies in your reaction to significant people giving you a neutral response. If you believe that you must have the approval of significant others, you will feel disturbed about receiving a neutral response because you are not getting the approval that you believe you need. However, if you believe that you must not be disapproved of by significant others, then you wouldn't feel disturbed about their neutral response to you because such a response does not constitute disapproval.

2 Having said this, you find it difficult to see the neutral responses of significant others to you as indicating neutrality. You tend to see them as disapproval. In addition, when others do disapprove of you, you tend to overestimate how much they disapprove of you and how long such disapproval will last.

3 When significant others disapprove of your behaviour, you think that this means that they disapprove of you as a person.

4 You base your self-worth on how significant people in your life view you.

5 You are highly sensitive to the moods of others and try to modify your behaviour to fit in with others so that they approve of you (or don't disapprove of you).

6 You think that if significant others disapprove of you (or don't approve of you) this must be your fault.

7 You would rather sacrifice your own best interests to gain the approval of significant others (or to avoid incurring their disapproval).

8 Whenever you think about doing the task over which you are procrastinating, you imagine significant others identifying what's wrong about what you are doing and disapproving of you.

In order to tackle approval-based procrastination it is important that you do the following:

1 Challenge the idea that you have to have the approval of significant others or that these others must not disapprove of you, using the methods outlined in the first part of this book (see chapter 5). Realize that while it is desirable to gain approval (or to avoid disapproval) it is not essential that you are approved (or not disapproved).

2 Recognize that while people who are significant to you are, in all probability, interested in what you do, they may well not be interested in you to the extent that you think they are. They may at times be neutral about what you do and how you do it. They are often preoccupied with themselves and are thinking of what they themselves are doing rather than what you are doing. When they do disapprove of you, realize that this is more fleeting than you think it is, in the same way as any disapproval of them that you experience is probably fleeting.

3 When significant others disapprove of your behaviour, acknowledge that this doesn't mean that they disapprove of you as a person. Even when they do, as I have shown above, this is in all probability time-limited.

4 If you base your self-worth on anything, base it on things that don't change about you, i.e. your aliveness, humanity, fallibility and uniqueness, rather than on how significant people in your life view you.

5 Be aware of the moods of others, but don't scrutinize them for a read-out of how they are feeling. Resolve not to change your behaviour to fit in with others. Risk receiving their disapproval and accept yourself if you get it. As you develop this attitude, show significant others examples of your work and accept yourself for any criticism that you get.

6 If significant others disapprove of you (or don't approve of you) this

may or may not be due to what you have done or not done. If it is due to something that you have done (for example), the important thing is that you take responsibility for what you have done, but do not blame yourself for your actions. In this case, strive to develop a philosophy of responsibility without blame. This involves you saying to yourself that you are the author of your behaviour that resulted in others disapproving of you, but this doesn't mean that you are a bad or worthless person for acting in the way that you did. Rather, recognize that you are the author of your behaviour, but this only proves that you are a fallible human being who has acted in an unfortunate manner. It does not prove that you are a bad or worthless person. Responsibility with blame, by contrast, involves you owning your behaviour *and* blaming or condemning yourself for acting in that way.

However, when a significant other disapproves of you for what you have done (or for what you have not done), this may reflect more on the other person's own views and attitudes than it does on your behaviour. To judge which is the case, ask yourself how a jury of twelve objective people would have viewed your behaviour. If the majority would not have disapproved of you for what you did (or did not do), then it is likely that the disapproval that you received at the hands of your significant other has more to do with them than it has to do with you and how you acted. Remember these points as you strive to overcome your chronic procrastination.

7 Don't sacrifice your own best interests to gain the approval of significant others (or to avoid incurring their disapproval). If you continue to do this you will undermine your attempts to acquire a healthy, flexible, non-demanding philosophy towards approval. One of the blocks you may encounter as you strive to give up self-sacrifice is that you may think you are being selfish. Realize that there is a difference between selfishness and enlightened self-interest. As I discussed in my book *Ten Steps to Positive Living* (Sheldon Press, 1994), selfishness involves you compulsively putting yourself first without due regard for the feelings and concerns of others. Enlightened self-interest, on the other hand, means that you are concerned with your own interests and with the interests of significant others, and that while most of the time you will put your own interests first with the interests of others a close second, some of the time you will put the interests of others before your own when their concerns are more pressing than your own. In brief, selfishness

involves you putting yourself first without due regard for the interests of others; self-sacrifice involves you putting others first without due regard for your own interests. Both of these positions are, as you can see, extreme positions. Enlightened self-interest, on the other hand, is a more flexible position. It involves you taking care of yourself so that at times you can take care of others. So if your procrastination is approval-based, then adopting a philosophy of enlightened self-interest will help you to overcome it.

8 Once you have made some progress in challenging and changing your belief that you must have the approval of significant others for what you have done, you will then begin to see that if you don't do perfectly well on the task in question, then you will get a range of reactions from other people in response to your task performance. Some will disapprove of you as a person, some will disapprove of what you have done but will not disapprove of you as a person, others will approve of you as a person, another group will approve of what you have done without thinking better of you as a person, and yet others will be neutral about what you have done. This contrasts with your views on this issue when you believe that you must be approved for what you do. When you have a dire need for the approval of others and you don't do well on the task under consideration, then you will tend to think that all significant others will disapprove of you as a person.

Thus, while your dire need for others' approval will tend to lead you to think only of others' disapproving of you should you put a foot wrong on the task – a mind-set that promotes procrastination – your full preference for receiving the approval of others will lead you to develop a balanced view with respect to the responses of others to your task performance – a mind-set that is more likely to help you to do the task at hand.

10
Dealing with Discomfort-based Procrastination

Discomfort-based procrastination occurs when you put off taking action that is in your best interests to take in order to maintain a sense of comfort, to get rid of feeling uncomfortable or to avoid experiencing a state of discomfort that you predict you will experience if you begin the task in question. However, the crucial ingredient that is at the core of discomfort-based procrastination is your unhealthy belief about discomfort/comfort.

Thus, when you are faced with beginning a task and you are in a state of comfort, the reason why you procrastinate is not because you are comfortable but because of your unhealthy belief about maintaining your comfortable state (e.g. 'I must continue to be comfortable and I can't bear making myself uncomfortable by starting the task in question').

Also, if you do decide to begin the task in question and you start to experience a sense of discomfort, you will tend to stop doing the task and put it off if you hold an unhealthy belief about the discomfort that you have begun to experience (e.g. 'I can't bear this discomfort. I have to get rid of it as quickly as possible').

Finally, if you predict that you will experience discomfort should you begin the task in question, your unhealthy belief about your predicted discomfort will lead to procrastination (e.g. 'If I begin the task and feel uncomfortable doing so, I can't bear that. I must not feel discomfort while doing the task'). It follows from the above that if you want to overcome your chronic specific or general procrastination, it is important that you first identify, challenge and change your unhealthy beliefs about losing your sense of comfort and experiencing a sense of discomfort, and second develop a set of healthy beliefs that involve you tolerating a loss of comfort and experiencing discomfort because it is in your best interests to do so. This latter point is important. I am not advocating that you develop a discomfort-tolerant philosophy just for the sake of it. Rather, I am advocating that you develop such a philosophy because it will help you to overcome your chronic procrastination problem and live a more effective life (assuming that you wish to do so).

Thus, when you are faced with beginning a task and you are in a state of comfort, you will be able to move from this state to a temporary state of discomfort – which normally accompanies beginning a task that is less pleasurable than that in which you have previously been engaged – if you hold a healthy belief about maintaining your comfortable state (e.g. 'I'd like to continue to be comfortable, but I don't have to do so. I can bear making myself uncomfortable, by starting the task in question, and it is worth it for me to do so').

Also, if you do decide to begin the task in question and you start to experience a sense of discomfort, you will continue doing the task rather than stopping it if you hold a healthy belief about the discomfort that you have begun to experience (e.g. 'I can bear this discomfort and I don't have to get rid of it as quickly as possible. I can stay with it because it is in my best interests to do so').

Finally, if you predict that you will experience discomfort should you begin the task in question, your healthy belief about your predicted discomfort will lead you to begin the task rather than to procrastinate (e.g. 'If I begin the task and feel uncomfortable doing so, I can bear that. I'd prefer not to feel discomfort while doing the task, but I do not have to be spared this experience. Also, it is worth it to me to do the task even though I am uncomfortable').

Once again I want to emphasize that your healthy beliefs on their own will not help you to overcome procrastination. But your healthy beliefs backed up by repeated action that is consistent with these beliefs will. For example, if you hold the following belief: 'If I begin the task and feel uncomfortable doing so, I can bear that. I'd prefer not to feel discomfort while doing the task, but I do not have to be spared this experience. Also it is worth it to me to do the task even though I am uncomfortable', but you do not begin the task in question, your continued procrastination will undermine your conviction in your healthy belief. In such a case, while you may be holding the new belief in your head, you are acting as if you believe its unhealthy alternative, i.e. 'If I begin the task and feel uncomfortable doing so, I can't bear that. I must not feel discomfort while doing the task.' In such instances, the belief that is backed up by action is strengthened and the belief that is not backed up by action is weakened. This is one of the most important principles of overcoming procrastination, and as such I am going to highlight it.

> The best way to overcome procrastination is to think healthily and act in ways that are consistent with this healthy thinking.

Let me take what I have said about discomfort-based procrastination and how to overcome it and apply it to common discomfort-related procrastination problems.

Inertia

When you operate according to the principle of inertia, you have a strongly felt tendency to continue doing what you are doing. Most often, inertia is taken to mean difficulty getting going. Thus, a typical scenario involves you lying in front of the television watching programmes that you have little interest in, knowing that you are wasting your time and that it would be a good idea to get up to do a task that is in your best interests to do, but you do not budge. Why? Because you are comfortable and won't make the transition from comfort (i.e. lying down) to discomfort (making the effort to get up and begin a task that may be unpleasant) even though you know in your head that your discomfort will be short-lived. You don't make the effort because you believe that you must not lose the comfort of the moment, and that experiencing the discomfort associated with getting up to get going will be too much for you.

If your chronic procrastination is largely inertia-based, it is important that you do two things. First, develop a healthy attitude towards comfort and discomfort. Prove to yourself that, while it may be undesirable for you to lose the comfort of the moment, there is no law which decrees that you must not give up feeling comfortable when it is in your interests to do so. Show yourself that it is difficult moving from comfort to discomfort, but just because it is difficult does not mean that it is too difficult to do so. You would undoubtedly do it if you smelt smoke in the next room, wouldn't you? Of course you would. This proves that it isn't *too* difficult. You would do it if it was worth it to you, and therefore it is important for you to bring to the forefront of your mind why making the transition from comfort to discomfort is worth your while.

Second, gain lots of practice at acting against your inertia. Deliberately seek out comfort, stay with it for a while and then force yourself up to get going, even though it is uncomfortable to do so. Such practice will really benefit you in the long run, as it will help you to break the inertia pattern and to show yourself that you can give up short-term comfort for long-term gain. Yes, I can hear you say, you know this. But, I retort, you only truly know it if you can do it.

The need for instant gratification

If you believe that you have to have what you want when you want it, you believe that you need instant gratification. This belief will make it very hard for you to begin a task that is in your own best interests to do when there are other, more attractive options open to you. Even if you begin work at the task in question, then your belief that you need immediate gratification will ensure that you soon switch to some other activity that has more immediate appeal. One of my clients, Brian, was a 20-year-old student at university who complained that he couldn't get any work done because people kept knocking at his door, asking him to join them for one appealing distraction or other when he was trying to get some studying done. When I asked him why he stopped work to go with his friends he stared at me with blank amazement. It was obvious why he went with his friends, he replied, because what they were offering was more enjoyable than work.

Let's face it, whenever you are faced with getting down to work on something that has limited appeal, but which is in your best interests to do (such as studying or getting your accounts in order), there is always something more enjoyable that you could be doing. And if you begin work at the task in question, there is always something more attractive on offer than what you are doing to tempt you away from your work. This is why, if you believe that you must have what you want when you want it and you want to overcome your long-standing procrastination problem, then you will have to develop a healthier perspective to dealing with being immediately gratified. As you can probably guess by now, there are two main ways of doing this. First, use all the techniques that I have discussed so far which are designed to help you to challenge your unhealthy belief, i.e. 'I must have what I want when I want it and I can't bear it when I don't get what I want immediately' and to adopt and strengthen its healthy alternative: 'I prefer to get what I want when I want, but I don't have to be immediately gratified. I can bear being so deprived and I will forgo immediate pleasures when it is in my longer-term interests to do so.'

67

Second, act, act and act again in ways that are consistent with this healthy belief. The more you do so, the more you will internalize a healthy belief about forgoing immediate pleasures. Doing so will help you to develop what is known as a philosophy of long-range hedonism. This means that you will strike a balance between engaging in short-term pleasures and forgoing these pleasures and working towards your longer-term goals. This flexible position is difficult to adopt, and for you to do so you will have to become more proficient at giving up your immediate pleasures.

The demand for instant achievement and quick solutions

Another form of discomfort intolerance is known as the demand for instant achievements and quick solutions. When you believe that you must be able to do whatever is in your best interests as quickly as possible, then you are likely to postpone beginning the task when you see, in advance, that it is reasonably complex and that you are not likely to be able to do it quickly. In addition, holding this unhealthy belief you may begin tackling some problem that you think will be quickly solved and give up as soon as it becomes apparent that you will not be able to solve the problem quickly.

As before, the best way to deal with procrastination that is underpinned by the demand for instant achievement and quick solutions is first to challenge the belief that you need to achieve things and solve problems quickly. That would be nice, I grant you, but why is it necessary? The answer is that it is not. If there was a law of the universe that decreed you had to solve problems and achieve things quickly, then you would. You would have to go along with such a law. Obviously, therefore, no such law exists, except, of course, in your head, which if you keep alive will maintain your chronic procrastination problem. So if you want to overcome rather than maintain this problem, stick with your healthy full preference: 'Yes, I would very much like to solve problems quickly and achieve things instantly, but I definitely don't have to do so. It's frustrating when tasks and problems take longer than I would like, but that, unfortunately, is life. Tough! I don't like it, but I can definitely lump it!'

If you will take this belief and resolve to act on it again repeatedly, you will raise your tolerance level by doing tasks and solving problems that don't yield to instant achievement and quick solutions respectively, and will begin to overcome your chronic procrastination problem to boot.

Waiting for effortless activity

If the previous type of discomfort-related procrastination involved you demanding quick results to your efforts, when you put off doing something until you can do it effortlessly you are demanding to be able to do things easily. While these two demands often go together (e.g. 'I have to do things quickly and easily') – and when they do they often lead to the most resistant forms of procrastination – they are in some ways different. Thus, if you demand to do things without making much effort, you may be prepared to engage in longer-term activity as long as you don't have to expend much energy in the process. If you are allergic to making an effort, you do need to challenge and change the belief that you have to do things easily and that it is terrible and intolerable if you have to really push yourself to get things done. It really is important that you change this belief, because there are precious few things in life that you can achieve effortlessly. So get used to expending some energy on those tasks that require it and are in your interests to do. Expending energy in all probability won't kill you. If it did, the human race would not have survived. Plenty of people make an effort and are rewarded by getting what they need to do done. Why do you have to be different? The answer is, plainly and simply put, *you don't!* Accepting and acting on this grim reality will help you to overcome your procrastination. Rebelling against it and trying to get others to do the work for you may help you in the short term, but it will maintain your chronic procrastination in the long term.

Mood-dominated action

The final type of discomfort-related procrastination that I will discuss is related to what those who suffer from it refer to as being 'in the mood'. If your procrastination is dominated by mood, you believe that you can't start an activity that is in your interests to do unless you are in the mood (or the right frame of mind) to do so. I encountered this phenomenon frequently when I counselled students at the University of Aston in Birmingham in the mid 1970s to the mid 1980s. About a month before their examinations began, hordes of students used to come for counselling, complaining about procrastination over their revision. Here is a typical exchange with a student suffering from mood-driven procrastination.

WINDY: OK, so why do you think you are putting off revising for your exams when, as you yourself have admitted, it is in your best interests to do so?

STUDENT: Because I don't feel like revising.

WINDY: When do you 'feel like' revising?

STUDENT: That's the trouble, doc, I never feel like revising.

WINDY: Do you 'feel like' getting your degree?

STUDENT: Oh, yes. I definitely want my degree.

WINDY: So it seems to me that you have a choice. Either you try to persuade the university to give you a degree, although, of course, they might not 'feel like' doing so unless you pass their exams, or you do what you don't 'feel like' doing in order to get what you 'feel like' getting.

STUDENT: Well, that's not much of a choice, is it? The University of Aston isn't going to give me a degree unless I pass my exams, are they?

WINDY: Well, you can ask them, but you're right, somehow I don't think that they are going to do that.

STUDENT: So, we're left with the other option. But how do I get myself into the mood to revise?

WINDY: That's your problem. You're trying to get yourself into the mood before you do something that you don't 'feel like' doing. The only way out of your dilemma is to begin to revise even when you're not in the mood to revise. Then, after a while, you stand a better chance of being in the mood to work than if you wait for the mood to strike you before you begin.

STUDENT: But don't I have to be in the mood to work before I work?

WINDY: Of course not. That's your major problem right there. You believe that you have to be in the mood to revise before revising. If that were true, nobody would revise. Now, it's true that it would be nice to be in the mood before you began to revise, but does it follow that you have to be?

STUDENT: I guess not.

WINDY: You guessed right. Now, if you put that new belief into practice, what would happen?

STUDENT: I'd revise even though I wasn't in the mood.

WINDY: And if you did so many times, some of the time you would get into the mood and some of the time you wouldn't, but you would revise anyway.

STUDENT: So is that all there is to it?

WINDY: If that's the only reason why you procrastinate, yes. However, you'll find that it's easier said than done. But [said with irony] you didn't come here expecting an easy solution, did you?

STUDENT: Well . . . I did, but I can see that I'm not going to get it.

WINDY: But I hope I've dispelled your notion that you have to be in the mood to revise before you revise.

STUDENT: You've certainly done that.

WINDY: So go off and practise, and then the university will 'feel like' giving you that degree . . . as long as you pass their lousy exams, that is.

This interchange demonstrates a number of points in considering and tackling mood-related procrastination. First, it is important to acknowledge that you don't have to be in the mood to tackle a task that is in your interests to tackle. Second, if you wait to get into the mood before you do something, then you may wait a very long time for this mood to come. Third, if you act according to the idea that you need to be in the mood or the right frame of mind before you do something, then you strengthen your conviction in this belief. Fourth, the best way to overcome mood-driven procrastination is by fully acknowledging the advantages, but not the necessity, of being in the mood before beginning a task that is in your interests to begin, and by acting repeatedly in ways that are consistent with this healthy belief; i.e. to do things that are in your interests to do when you don't feel like doing them. Finally, realize that if you follow the aforementioned principle

71

you will, at least some of the time, get into the mood after starting the task in question.

The reason why I have devoted so much space to discomfort-related procrastination is that it is very common. It can be the main reason why you put things off or it may accompany one or more of the other reasons for your procrastination problem. Whichever is the case, developing a philosophy of discomfort tolerance is a central feature of overcoming chronic procrastination, not only in the short term but in the longer term as well.

11

Dealing with Worry-based Procrastination

If you experience worry-based procrastination you tend to display some or all of the following:

1 You hold an unhealthy awfulizing belief about what might go wrong if you attempt the task in question.

2 You tend to overestimate what might go wrong if you attempt the task and underestimate what might go right.

3 You believe that you have to be confident before you attempt the task.

4 You tend to have low confidence in your ability to do the task.

5 You are unsure about how best to do the task in question and believe that you have to have such certainty. Consequently, you tend to suffer from indecisiveness.

6 You tend to rely too much on other people's opinions about what to do and how best to do it. You ask a number of people for their opinions on this matter and become confused when different people give you different opinions. You don't attempt the task because you believe that you have to know for sure which is the right task to do first and how best to do it. Thus, you believe that there is a right way to do the task in question and a right order in which to do several tasks, and hold that you have to discover these right answers before you begin anything.

7 You tend to resist change and go for the familiar even if this means procrastinating.

In order to tackle worry-based procrastination, I suggest that you do the following:

1 Keep challenging your awfulizing beliefs and show yourself that while it would be bad if things went wrong as a result of you attempting the task in question, it is not the end of the world if this happens. Developing an anti-awfulizing philosophy is perhaps the most important ingredient in overcoming worry-based chronic procrastination. Once you have made progress at this, you are better placed to see that you can learn from what goes wrong.

2 In addition, developing an anti-awfulizing philosophy towards what might go wrong as a result of doing the task in question will help you to see that in reality there is a balance between what might go wrong and what might go right.

3 Challenge your unhealthy belief that you have to be confident before you attempt the task in question. Doing so will help you to see more clearly that perhaps the best way to develop task confidence is to do things unconfidently at first and to learn from your errors as you do so.

4 Realizing that you don't have to be confident at something before you attempt it and acting in ways that are consistent with this healthy belief will increase your level of confidence in your ability to do the task.

5 Challenge the unhealthy belief that you have to be sure about how best to do a task before you do it. Get used to taking sensible risks and tolerate the discomfort that accompanies such risk-taking. Taking action consistent with this healthy belief will help you to dispel indecisiveness.

6 Stop asking other people for their opinions about what to do and how best to do it. Get used to taking independent action even though this is unfamiliar and uncomfortable. Realize that there are a number of ways of tackling a given task and a variety of orders in which you can tackle several tasks. Even if there is a best way and a best order, give up the unhealthy demand that you have to find it before taking action. Get used to encouraging and supporting yourself and decrease your reliance on gaining encouragement and support from others.

7 Recognize that while you may prefer familiarity and dislike change, you don't always have to have the former and avoid the latter. Again, practise tolerating the discomfort that change inevitably brings as you overcome your chronic procrastination.

8 Seek out people who are self-reliant and who take action with due concern but without undue worry, and learn from them.

12

Dealing with Autonomy-based Procrastination

If you suffer from autonomy-based procrastination, you put off tasks that are in your best interests to do because other people require or want you to do them and you see their requests or demands as encroachments on your autonomy, a state you hold very dear indeed. This type of procrastination is characterized by some or all of the following:

1 You hold the unhealthy belief that you must have autonomy in your life, meaning the freedom to determine your own direction free from the requirements of others. If others require you to do something, you tend to defy them, even if doing so is not in your best interests. Viewed from this perspective, procrastination is seen as an act of defiance designed to restore a sense of balance; in this case, it restores your sense of autonomy.

2 You tend to believe that if you do what others want or require of you, you are a weak, spineless person even if you want to do the task in question and/or it is in your own best interests to do so. You tend to base your self-worth on your autonomy.

3 You are highly sensitive to encroachments on your freedom or autonomy and tend to view even the mildest requests of others as burdens to be resisted. You also often think that others are on your back even in the absence of supportive evidence.

4 You have a hostile attitude to others who want or require you to do things, even when it is in your best interests to do them. You believe that others must leave you alone to do what you want to do, in the way that you want to do it and when you want to do it. You then see putting a task off as a way of getting back at these others. Thwarting others thus becomes more important to you than doing what is in your best interests to do. You are thus seen as 'cutting off your nose to spite your face'.

5 You detest rules that you disagree with and think that they absolutely should not apply to you.

6 You detest authority and find ways to resist it. If you are scared to challenge authority openly, you find covert ways of doing so and can be said to be acting in a passive-aggressive manner.

7 You prefer working on your own and have a strong dislike of

working in teams. If you do have to work in a team you see compromise as weakness which has to be resisted.

I recommend the following ways to overcome autonomy-based procrastination:

1 Powerfully and repeatedly challenge the unhealthy belief that you must have autonomy in your life. Realize that autonomy is important to you, but is not the be-all and end-all of your life. This is perhaps the central ingredient in overcoming autonomy-based procrastination.

2 See clearly that if you seek autonomy by procrastinating on tasks that others want or require you to do that are, in fact, in your best interests to do, then you are allowing yourself to be controlled by them and are not truly autonomous. If you had true autonomy then you would be able to do something because *you* determine that it is in your best interests to do it even though others want or even order you to do it. Adopting this position would help you to focus more on what is in your best interests and less on what others want or require you to do.

3 Give up the idea that you are a weak, spineless person if you do what others want or require you to do. Even if going along with others is a weakness (which it often isn't when doing the task in question is in your best interests), then doing it only means that you are a fallible human being who has strengths and weaknesses. If you were a weak person you could only act weakly in life, which is hardly likely to be true. Developing a philosophy of unconditional self-acceptance will help you to stop proving how strong and autonomous you are by defying others. For more information on how to develop unconditional self-acceptance, I recommend that you consult my book entitled *How to Accept Yourself* (Sheldon Press, 1999).

4 Once you have started to develop a flexible attitude towards autonomy and have begun to accept yourself as a person with strengths and weaknesses who doesn't have to keep proving to yourself how strong and autonomous you are, then you will become far less sensitive to encroachments on your freedom or autonomy. You will begin to distinguish between fair and unfair requests and demands from others. You will also begin to see others more objectively and recognize that, while some people may get on your back unfairly, it is more often the case that others want you to do things for perfectly legitimate reasons.

5 Identify and keep challenging your unhealthy hostile beliefs that others must leave you alone to do what you want to do, in the way that you want to do it and when you want to do it. They are not bad people for wanting you to do things that you may not want to do. Rather, they are fallible human beings who may be acting unfairly towards you, but more often than not they have good reasons for wanting you to do things a certain way. This healthy attitude will help you to stop putting a task off to get back at others, since you will no longer experience a need to defy them. Your focus will be more on doing what is in your interests to do than on thwarting others.

6 As you develop these healthy and flexible attitudes, you may still dislike rules that you disagree with, but are far less likely to think that they absolutely should not apply to you. These healthy beliefs will also help you to assert yourself appropriately when you are faced with unfair rules and will tend to decrease markedly your urge to act passive-aggressively.

7 In addition, as you adopt the above beliefs you may still dislike authority, but only when you see that it is being misused. In such cases you will assert yourself when it is in your best interests to do so. However, you will also begin to see that authority can be used wisely and humanely, and that such forms of authority need to be supported rather than indiscriminantly resisted.

8 Developing these beliefs may not change your preference to work on your own and you still may not like working in teams. But if you do have to work in a team you will learn that compromise is more often than not a strength rather than a weakness and can lead to effective team performance. Procrastination, on the other hand, will help neither you nor the team in which you are working.

13
Dealing with Crisis-based Procrastination

By crisis-based procrastination, I mean a situation where you put off until the very last minute doing something that is in your best interests to do. While most forms of procrastination are crisis-based to some degree, when your procrastination is defined by its crisis-based nature the following are its basic features:

- When faced with doing something that is in your interests to do but which you find unpleasant, you go from long periods of inactivity to intense activity conducted at the very last minute. It is as if you only have two speeds: stop and breakneck speed.
- You easily become bored and dread doing things methodically and persistently. Thus, you tend to have a marked philosophy of discomfort intolerance.
- You tend to get a buzz from living on the edge.
- You tend to think that being under stress or being anxious is a productive motivator.
- You frequently use the built-in excuse that goes along with crisis-based procrastination: 'I would have done better if I hadn't done it in a rush at the last minute.'
- You tend to dramatize situations.
- Your crisis-based procrastination tends to be reinforced by the fact that you often manage to do things at the last minute. Thus, you are ambivalent about changing your last-minute work pattern.

In order to overcome crisis-based procrastination, you need to do the following:

1 Do a cost-benefit analysis of doing things at the very last minute versus doing things earlier. See clearly that while you may think that doing things at the very last minute has paid off for you, in reality you are more likely to do better if you give yourself more time to to tasks.
2 Develop a range of speeds at which you do tasks rather than the two you have habitually employed (i.e. stop and breakneck speed). Get used to working steadily. You may not like this speed, but it is an

additional speed to your gauge and one that is very helpful for tasks that you can't do at the very last minute.

3 Challenge and change your unhealthy belief that you cannot stand the tedium of working methodically and persistently at something. Really work to raise your level of discomfort tolerance on this issue and force yourself to start things much earlier than you are accustomed to doing. You won't feel natural doing so – this will come much later – but it will pay off in the longer term.

4 Seek out excitement and 'buzzes' in areas of life in which these states are healthy rather than unhealthy.

5 Accept the fact that the reason you tend to think that being under stress or being anxious are productive motivators is because you have trained yourself to get going only when you experience such states. Get used to doing things when you don't 'feel' like it and realize that some of the time you will become motivated in the course of working in this way. Appreciate that being under pressure does get you going, but not necessarily effectively. A headless chicken gets going, but is not that productive in its activity! Identify and act on other motivations apart from stress and anxiety.

6 Don't use the built-in excuse that goes along with crisis-based procrastination: 'I would have done better if I hadn't done it in a rush at the last minute.' Show yourself why this is an excuse and not a valid reason. Instead, remind yourself that you probably will do better if you start earlier, and if you don't, this does not prove you are incompetent. Rather, it proves that you are a fallible human being who didn't do as well as you wanted on this occasion, but that you can learn from this experience to do better next time.

7 Tolerate the boredom of doing uninteresting tasks that are in your interests to do and actively look for and focus on any interesting components of these tasks.

8 Realize that you are not a boring person if you begin the task with plenty of time in hand. Rather, you are a complex, fallible human being with many different facets, including being sensible and dramatic.

9 Gain control of your tendency to dramatize situations. Use this tendency in non self-defeating situations. Additionally, seek out areas of life where you can develop your capacity to be peaceful and serene.

14

Dealing with Other Forms of Procrastination

In this chapter, I will cover five lesser-known types of procrastination.

Dealing with identification-based procrastination

If you suffer from identification-based procrastination, you put off doing something that reminds you of somebody of whom you do not wish to be reminded. Here, procrastination enables you to escape the identification that you would make if you did the task. However, it is not just the fact of the identification that leads you to procrastinate; rather, it is the belief that you hold about the identification. Let me give you an example. Judy has great difficulty keeping her financial accounts in order. Every time she thinks about doing this work she is reminded of her mother, whom she dislikes, who is good at dealing with money. In Judy's mind, doing her accounts on time means that she is like her mother. Now, Judy holds the unhealthy belief that she must not be like her mother, and that if she is this means she is a nasty person (which is how she views her mother). Since she doesn't want to be a nasty person in her own eyes, she has to be unlike her mother, and in this case this means that she has to put off doing her accounts. In order for Judy to overcome her identification-based procrastination, she needs to give up her demand that she must not be anything like her mother and accept herself if she is. This will enable her to do her financial accounts and make a good job of them.

So, if you suffer from identification-based procrastination, you need to challenge your demand that you must not share any characteristic with the person whom you dislike and then do the task in question. Recognize that both you and the other person are competent at the task and that you can accept yourself for being like that person in this respect.

Dealing with memory-triggered procrastination

In memory-triggered procrastination, you put off doing something that is in your best interests to do because doing the task triggers a memory about which you awfulize. For example, Mary put off cooking for friends to whom she owed hospitality because if she had a dinner party she would remember her cooking being criticized by her ex-husband, a situation she regarded as terrible. Her counsellor helped Mary overcome her culinary procrastination by encouraging her to take the horror out of being criticized. Mary was then able to enjoy having friends around for food.

Thus, the best way to overcome memory-triggered procrastination is for you to challenge and change your awfulizing belief about the remembered experience before doing the task in question.

Dealing with overcommitment-based procrastination

In overcommitment-based procrastination, you put off doing something because you have too much work to do. Your procrastination is thus a logical consequence of overstretching yourself (see Chapter 3). Your real problem here is that you have taken on too much work because you have a problem saying no. One major reason why you find it difficult to turn down work is that should you do so, you would experience unhealthy guilt. This type of guilt is based on the belief that you are a bad person for letting others down. In order to overcome your feelings of guilt you have to challenge this idea and show yourself that while it may be bad to let others down, you are not a bad person for doing so. Rather, you are a fallible human who doesn't have to meet the expectations of others. In doing so, it is important that you develop a philosophy of enlightened self-interest. This involves you committing yourself primarily to fulfilling your own interests and secondarily to fulfilling the interests of others. Some of the time you will put the interests of others over your own, but you do not do so as a matter of course. This will enable you to say no and allow you not to overcommit yourself.

A second major reason why you find it hard to turn down doing a task that is not in your interests to take on is because you think that if you do so, then your work will soon dry up. This latter inference is distorted and is based on your unhealthy belief that you must not let any opportunity slip. If you challenge and change this belief, then you will realize that you are engaging in black-and-white thinking and that, in reality, if you turn down one or several pieces of work, it does not follow that all your work will dry up. Rather, you will still have work to do and have a more manageable work load. This work load will mean that you will have the time to do everything that you need to do.

Dealing with narcissistic-based procrastination

In narcissistic-based procrastination, you put off doing something that is in your best interests to do, because you think that doing the task in question is beneath you and you believe that you must not do tasks which are beneath you. In this type of procrastination, you are acutely aware of your status and you base your self-esteem on being in high-status positions. If your procrastination is narcissistically based, you need to challenge the idea that you must not do things that you consider are beneath you, and recognize that doing these things does not diminish you as a person. Make your self-esteem unconditional rather than conditionally based on being in high-status positions. Show yourself that being in such positions has its advantages but is not the be-all and end-all of life, and if it is in your best interests to do a low status task, push yourself to do it.

Dealing with procrastination as an interpersonal ploy

When procrastination is employed as an interpersonal ploy, you put off doing something in order to get a response from others. In my experience, the most common response that is sought is for another person to do the task for you. In other words, procrastination here is a form of dependency. As I have discussed this form of procrastination more extensively earlier in this book (see pp. 22–24), I will confine myself to discussing how to tackle it.

First, you need to understand which response you are trying to elicit from others when you procrastinate.

Second, you need to decide that it is in your best interests to overcome this form of procrastination and to give up the perceived advantages that it is designed to get for you. Here you may wish to use the cost-benefit analysis form described earlier (see pp. 8–15).

Third, you need to identify the unhealthy beliefs that underpin your behaviour. Ask yourself the question: In getting someone to do the task for me, what am I demanding? When you procrastinate in order to get another person to do the task for you, you may hold one or more of the following unhealthy beliefs:

- I must be spared the effort of doing this task. Others must do it for me.
- I must do the task well. Since I don't think I can do it well, someone must do it for me.

- Other people know how to do things better than me. So I might as well let them do it for me, because I have to have their help.

Fourth, challenge and change these beliefs using the methods described earlier in the book. The healthy alternatives to the above-mentioned unhealthy beliefs are:

- I'd like to be spared the effort of doing this task, but I don't have to be so spared. Others don't have to do it for me. I can do it myself.
- I'd like to do the task well, but it isn't essential for me to do so. Although I don't think I can do it well, I'll do it and see, and learn from my errors. It is not necessary or even desirable for someone else to do it for me.
- Other people may know how to do things better than me, but I'll do the task myself because this is the only way for me to learn how to do it. I don't need other people to take over for me.

Finally, act in ways that are consistent with these healthy beliefs. This means doing the task in question on your own without recourse to help from others. Only when you have struggled with the task for a long time without profit should you ask for help. Even then, ask others to show you how to do the task rather than to do it for you.

PART 3
Other Techniques

15

A Smorgasbord of Other
Anti-procrastination Methods

So far in this book I have discussed what I consider to be the core of procrastination, i.e. the unhealthy beliefs that you hold which lead you to put off tasks that are in your best interests to do. My view is that unless you first develop a set of healthy anti-procrastination beliefs, then any more practical methods that you try to employ will only lead to short-lived results. This is why I have discussed changing your beliefs before considering the many practical tips that exist to help you overcome your chronic procrastination. Think of changing your beliefs as laying good solid foundations before you build a house. Not that I am arguing that you must always start with changing your procrastination-related beliefs before using these other methods. This would be inflexible and go against everything I teach about developing good mental health. But I do argue that whenever you can and whenever it is feasible to do so, start with changing these beliefs. Put another way, I am suggesting that overcoming procrastination is often best done by first addressing your unhealthy beliefs and then using a range of practical methods, but that there are exceptions to this principle. What follows, then, is a 'smorgasbord' of practical and psychological methods for you to sample after (in most cases) you have made progress in developing an anti-procrastination philosophy.

Don't label yourself as a procrastinator

If you label yourself as *a* procrastinator, then you will find it harder to overcome your chronic procrastination problem than if you do not label your entire self with your problem. For if you are *a* procrastinator then you will tend to continue to procrastinate, whereas if you regard yourself as a person with a procrastination problem who has the capacity to overcome this problem, then you will increase your chances of doing just that.

Accept yourself as a person who has a problem with procrastination

Similarly, it is important that you do not depreciate yourself for procrastinating. In my experience as a counsellor, people who do not depreciate themselves for procrastinating and accept themselves as fallible human beings who have a procrastination problem are more likely to overcome this problem than those who put themselves down for their problem by regarding themselves, for example, as weak, pathetic or incompetent. Depreciating yourself for procrastinating leads to you becoming preoccupied with how weak, pathetic and incompetent you are and takes you away from dealing effectively with this problem in the first place, whereas accepting yourself for having this problem helps to focus your energy on dealing with the factors that lead you to procrastinate.

Overcoming guilt about procrastination

People who have a chronic procrastination problem are often plagued with feelings of guilt, which interfere with them overcoming this particular problem as well as giving them a second problem (i.e. guilt). For example, if, as a result of your chronic procrastination problem, you consider that you have let others down or acted unethically (e.g. by cheating or plagiarizing the work of another) and feel guilty about these things, then your feelings of guilt will stop you from addressing your procrastination as effectively as you will be able to do if you experienced remorse but not guilt about such events. As I have shown in detail in my book *Overcoming Guilt* (Sheldon Press, 1994), the ABCs of guilt and remorse (the healthy alternative to guilt) are as follows:

Guilt

A (Activating event):   Doing something wrong
Failing to do the right thing
Hurting or letting down others

B (Belief):   Demand
Self-depreciation belief

C (Consequence):   Guilt

Remorse

A (Activating event):	Doing something wrong Failing to do the right thing Hurting or letting down others
B (Belief):	Full preference Self-acceptance belief
C (Consequence):	Remorse

Once you experience remorse rather than guilt you will come to terms with what happened at A, make appropriate amends and get on with the business of overcoming procrastination. It is important to note that the best way to overcome guilt is first to assume temporarily that what you did or didn't do or what happened at A was true, and then to challenge and change your unhealthy beliefs before going back to reconsider the accuracy of your inferences at A. I suggest this order because if you consider the accuracy of your inferences of what happened at A before challenging your unhealthy beliefs at B, your feelings of guilt will cloud your judgement and you will arrive at a biased conclusion.

While I have concentrated on guilt here, I do appreciate that other emotional problems often accompany procrastination. Space precludes a detailed exploration of all these problems, but here is a list of the most frequently occurring of such problems and appropriate reading suggestions (all published by Sheldon Press): anger (*Overcoming Anger* by Windy Dryden, 1996); shame (*Overcoming Shame*, by Windy Dryden, 1997); anxiety (*Overcoming Anxiety*, by Windy Dryden, 2000) and depression (*Think Your Way to Happiness* by Windy Dryden and Jack Gordon, 1990).

Dealing with 'pseudo-work'

'Pseudo-work' is the name I give when you engage in activities that at first sight seem like work, but on closer inspection are really delaying tactics. Such activities are related to actual work on a task, but are not in fact an intrinsic part of task activity. They are most often tasks that prepare the ground for task activity (e.g. sharpening pencils, tidying one's work space, cleaning work surfaces, etc.). Doing such activities is a good idea, but if you find that you are spending an inordinate amount of time on them then you are engaging in 'pseudo-work'.

A SMORGASBORD OF OTHER ANTI-PROCRASTINATION METHODS

Engaging in 'pseudo-work' gives you the impression that you are working and not procrastinating, but in reality you are engaged in a subtle form of procrastination. How can you tell if engaging in preparatory activities is 'pseudo-work'? You are engaging in 'psuedo-work' if:

- doing the activity takes longer than can be reasonably expected;
- you do this activity over and over again;
- you engage in three or more of such activities on any one occasion.

You need to be honest with yourself in identifying 'pseudo-work' (including reading books on overcoming procrastination!) as a procrastination ploy, but once you have done so you can use the methods I have already covered in this book to tackle your procrastination.

Dealing with distractions

People who have a chronic procrastination problem often complain about being distracted by their environment. I distinguish between two types of distraction: those within your control and those outside of your control. People who procrastinate often overestimate the number of distractions that are outside of their control and underestimate the number that are within their control. For example, do you complain about being interrupted by the phone? Then unplug it and, if necessary, get an answer machine and turn the volume down. Do people knock on your door, interrupting your concentration? Then put a 'Do not Disturb' sign on your door. Do the neighbours play loud music? Then ask them nicely to turn it down, wear ear plugs or go to the library.

All of the distractions that I have mentioned have been considered by my clients to be out of their control, yet in reality are in their control. If distractions are out of your control and you cannot change your working environment, then train yourself first to undisturb yourself about these distractions and then work as best you can in their wake. You can often do a little work in the presence of such distractions, which is better than doing no work at all.

Dealing with grasshopperism

By grasshopperism, I mean failing to get anything substantial done because you jump from activity to activity. If you suffer from grasshopperism, it is very likely that you have a low tolerance for boredom and move from task to task when you begin to feel bored.

The only real way of dealing with grasshopperism is to raise your tolerance level for boredom and show yourself both in thought and in deed that while being bored is unpleasant, it is a tolerable experience which is worth tolerating because you want to get the task done. If you raise your tolerance level for boredom and stay with feeling bored while continuing to do the task in question, you will discover that you tend to overestimate vastly how boring the task actually is, particularly when you stay with it and don't put it off. When you have raised your tolerance level for boredom, by all means look for ways of making mundane tasks more interesting. Most people reverse this order, but if you do this you do not deal with the core of grasshopperism, which is your perceived inability to tolerate boredom.

Dealing with behavioural excesses

Sometimes people with a chronic procrastination problem engage in various behavioural excesses (e.g. drinking and overeating) to forget their problem. When this occurs, the person soon develops a second problem more serious than the original procrastination problem. If you think you are beginning to engage in escapist behaviour to excess, then it is important that you address the main reason for this problem which is reflected in an unhealthy belief about your procrastination problem. The way you do this is as follows. First, identify how you honestly feel about having a procrastination problem. Second, identify what you are most disturbed about with respect to this problem. Third, identify the unhealthy beliefs that you have about this factor. Finally, challenge and change these unhealthy beliefs and replace them with healthy beliefs. You will then be in a better state to tackle the reasons why you procrastinate in the first place. If, however, your behavioural excess is out of control, then please see your doctor and ask for an appropriate referral to deal with this escalating problem.

Dealing with excuses or rationalizations

People who have a chronic procrastination problem are experts at coming up with a thousand and one 'good reasons' why they could not possibly have done what was in their best interests to do. The problem is that in the vast majority of cases, these 'good reasons' are nothing of the kind. They are excuses or rationalizations. Albert Ellis and William

Knaus have identified some of the most common, along with suggested counters:

● 'I need to feel under pressure before I can get down to work'
(Counter: 'I've trained myself to operate according to this principle, but I don't need pressure to do work')

● 'I'll wait until I know I can do the job properly'
(Counter: 'I don't need to know this before I start and I don't have to do it properly')

● 'It's not awful if I don't do it'
(Counter: 'True, but this isn't a reason not to start')

● 'I don't really want to do it'
(Counter: 'True, but the point is not what I want to do, but what I want to have done. If it is in my interests to do the task then I can do it even if I don't want to do it')

● 'I'll wait until I'm in the mood'
(Counter: 'I may wait a long time before I'm in the mood. I can do the task even though I am not in the mood to do it')

● 'If I do the task then I may miss out on things that I'll never get the chance to experience'
(Counter: 'I'll probably get the chance later to do these things, but even if I don't there is no law to say that I must not miss out on things')

● 'Circumstances stopped me from doing it'
(Counter: 'Unlikely. I stopped myself from doing it and I don't have to continue doing so')

● 'Nobody cares if I do it or not'
(Counter: 'Even if this is true, I care since it is in my interests to do it')

The best way to deal with rationalizations and excuses is to identify them, counter them as in the above examples and then act against them by doing the task in question.

Dealing with distorted inferences

If you have a chronic procrastination problem, the chances are that apart from having unhealthy beliefs, other aspects of your thinking are distorted too. In Rational Emotive Behaviour Therapy, we distinguish between two different types of thinking: beliefs and inferences. Inferences are hunches about reality which may be accurate or inaccurate, whereas beliefs are evaluations about reality. An example will make this clear. Let's suppose that you are procrastinating on a task that is in your interests to do. I ask you why you are putting off this task and you reply: 'Because I won't do it very well and it will be terrible if I don't.'

Using the ABC method we have:

A = Inference: Predicting that I will not do the task very well.

B = Belief (in this case unhealthy): 'It will be terrible if I don't do the task very well.'

C = Procrastination.

In this example, you are making an inference at A that you will not do the task very well and you are evaluating that inference at B in that you think it would be terrible if you don't do the task very well. Now the line I have taken in this book is that beliefs determine whether or not you procrastinate, not inferences. Thus, if you believed that it would be bad, but not terrible, if you did not do the task very well, you would be more likely to begin it because this anti-awfulizing belief would then help you to see more clearly than your awfulizing belief that it is in your interests to do the task. This is why I have suggested throughout this book that changing your unhealthy beliefs to healthy beliefs is a priority if you wish to overcome your chronic procrastination problem.

However, it could also be true that your inference is distorted. In this case there may be a very good chance of doing the task very well, and you are inferring that you won't do it well. Thinking clearly here will also help you to stop putting off the task in question. It is for this reason that, after you have challenged and changed your unhealthy beliefs, it is a good idea to inspect your inferences in case they are distorted.

How can you deal with your distorted inferences? I suggest the following steps, which should be done in writing on a piece of paper:

1 Inspect your inference to see if it is distorted. Is your inference an example of black-and-white thinking or are you making unrealistically negative predictions? Are you overestimating the difficulty of the task and underestimating your ability to do it? If so, your inference is distorted, so write it down on your piece of paper.

2 Stand back and ask yourself what evidence there is to support your inference and what evidence there is to contradict it. Do this in writing on the same piece of paper.

3 Ask yourself: 'What alternative ways of viewing the same situation are there?' Brainstorm as many possibilities as you can think of.

4 Look for evidence for and against these alternatives.

5 Stand back and choose the alternative that seems the most plausible.

While I recommend that you inspect your inferences after changing your unhealthy beliefs, there may be occasions when you may find reversing this order more profitable. Rational Emotive Behaviour Therapy is a flexible approach to counselling and sanctions departures from its preferred practice, if there are good reasons for these departures.

Develop problem-solving skills

Some people's chronic procrastination is exacerbated by their poor problem-solving skills. When they come to tackle the task in question they put it off again because they don't know how to use problem-solving skills to help them do the task. As I showed in my book *Ten Steps to Positive Living* (Sheldon Press, 1994), there are nine stages in the problem-solving sequence. Here are these nine stages:

1 Identify the problem to be tackled as clearly and as unambiguously as you can.

2 Set realistic, achievable, specific goals. These may be divided into short-term and long-term goals.

3 List all the possible ways of solving the problem.

4 List the pros and cons of each alternative.

5 Choose from your list the best alternative.

6 Plan how to implement this alternative, deciding on the steps you need to take to do this. Making a written step-by-step plan at this point is particularly useful.

7 Make a commitment to implement your chosen solution, specifying when, where and how you are going to do it.

8 After you have implemented your chosen solution, sit down and review what progress you have made towards your goal. At this point, decide what further steps you need to take in order to achieve your objective.

9 Evaluate the outcome of your chosen solution and decide whether other courses of action are necessary.

Again, the best time to use these skills is after you have challenged and changed your unhealthy beliefs that underpin your procrastination problem, but, as with correcting your distorted inferences, sometimes you will do so before working on belief change.

Develop a work schedule that suits you

I recently met a colleague, also a writer, and we discussed our respective work schedules. We are both prolific authors but have strikingly different work schedules. He works for long stretches of time in his study, mostly in the morning, and rarely works beyond 2 p.m., while I work in short bursts on my portable word-processor, mainly when I am travelling. We have both chosen a work schedule that suits us. I would struggle to work effectively according to his work schedule, and similarly he would struggle to work effectively under mine. So when you have made progress at developing an anti-procrastination philosophy, choose a work schedule that suits you – not other people, but you. Doing so will help you to overcome your chronic procrastination problem.

Modify your physical environment

Some people who have a chronic procrastination problem attempt to work in an environment which serves to discourage them from working. One of my clients preferred to work in a clean and tidy environment, but had not cleaned or tidied her study in two years. After she had made progress at developing an anti-procrastination strategy, she still tended to shy away from work because of the state of her office. Once she had spent three days cleaning the room thoroughly and tidying it up, then her working environment helped her to overcome her procrastination problem.

Once again, I wish to stress that what is a suitable physical working environment for one person may well be a work turn-off for another. So choose to work in an environment that suits you. It won't solve your procrastination problem on its own, but it will definitely help you along this path.

95

Assert yourself with saboteurs

If you have a chronic procrastination problem which you genuinely wish to overcome, I suggest that you explain to people what you are trying to do and enlist their support. Generally, people will be happy to help you, but sometimes one or two may consciously or more often unconsciously attempt to sabotage your efforts. In such cases, it is important that you assert yourself with these people and do two things. First, do not agree to put off working on your task if they suggest that you do so, and second, ask them firmly not to bother you. If this doesn't work you may need to break off contact with such people until you have done the task in question.

Henry, for example, was a DIY enthusiast who had a long history of procrastination. One day he made the decision to overcome this problem, as he could see that all the unfinished jobs around the house were beginning to put a strain on his marriage. Henry made good progress at tackling his problem and told his friends not to contact him for two weeks as he attempted to catch up on months of work. All but two of his friends did this. The others kept on tempting Henry to go out with them. Henry told both firmly not to do this and one agreed, but the other didn't and kept ignoring Henry's firmly expressed requests. So, Henry told this person that he did not want to see him until the house was completely finished. You will not be surprised to learn that this person also had a procrastination problem and couldn't stand the idea that Henry was doing something constructive about his problem when he wasn't.

Utilize a reward system

As I discussed earlier, one of the major reasons why people procrastinate is that they are not prepared to delay gratification. They put off difficult or unpleasant tasks that are in their interests to do and opt instead to do more immediately pleasurable things. If this applies to you, you may find it helpful to reward yourself for doing the task that you have previously put off. Thus, after you have worked on the task for an hour, for example, reward yourself with a cup of tea or coffee, and once you have finished the task altogether treat yourself with a trip to the cinema. Using rewards is helpful in two ways. First, they help to sustain your work on the task in question. In other words, they give you something to look forward to. Second, rewards tend to increase your future participation in rewarded activity. Thus, they make it more likely that you will do unpleasant tasks that are in your best interests to do in the future. Remember that it is important that you reward yourself *after* you have done the activity. When you procrastinate, you reward yourself *before* you do the task.

Penalize yourself if necessary

While rewards can be helpful in the ways just mentioned, some people are more receptive to penalties. When you employ penalties to encourage you to do something that is in your best interests to do rather than put off, select a penalty and resolve to apply it to yourself if you do not do the task within a reasonable time period agreed with yourself. If you do the task, you do not, of course, have to apply the penalty. Penalties may be mild (e.g. doing the washing up or agreeing not to watch your favourite TV programme) or severe (e.g. sending a sizeable monetary donation to a cause that you oppose). Severe penalties tend to work best for particularly intractable procrastination problems. Of course, penalties will only work when you actually apply them if you continue to procrastinate, but only use them after you have understood why you have been procrastinating and have begun to adopt an anti-procrastination philosophy. Also, don't use penalties that will harm others or yourself in any significant way. Thus, don't say that you will leave your job if you continue to procrastinate. Finally, the judicious conjoint use of rewards *and* penalties can be a particularly powerful way of overcoming chronic procrastination.

Allocate more time than the task will take

If you have a problem with procrastination, one of the rationalizations that you may use for postponing action is that you have plenty of time to do the task in question. However, if you are serious in overcoming your procrastination problem then it is important that you allow for the possibility that things may go wrong. This is why I recommend that you allocate more time to doing a task than it will realistically take. Use this time wisely and get used to doing things well before the deadline. Then you can use this spare time enjoying yourself.

A selection of practical tips for overcoming procrastination

I have not devoted much space in this book to a discussion of practical tips for overcoming procrastination because I don't think that such tips help you in the long term to overcome chronic procrastination. However, since these tips can be useful after you have made some progress in developing an anti-procrastination philosophy, they are worth considering. Here, then, are fifteen useful practical tips for overcoming procrastination.

1 Break the task down into bite-sized chunks.
2 Do something else and, once you have gained momentum, switch to the task that you have been putting off.
3 Use reminders.
4 Plan to spend five minutes on the task and then go on. Do five more minutes, possibly after a minute's break. Continue in this vein until you have done the task.
5 Do the task as soon as you think of it.
6 Allocate a set time for doing tasks that you 'feel like' putting off.
7 Mix with people who don't procrastinate, and follow their example.
8 Enlist the help of others to help you (but not to do the task for you).
9 Act as if you don't procrastinate.
10 Use bits of time on the task.
11 Identify the best time for task activity (e.g. when you have most energy) and do it then.
12 Do the most unpleasant or most difficult thing that you have to do immediately to get it out of the way.
13 Monitor your urges to put things off and act against them every time you identify them.
14 Picture yourself doing the task and then follow this in reality.
15 Use paradoxical intention. Every time you feel the urge to procrastinate, strive to do so to the best of your ability. This often helps when your problem is that you force yourself to do the task without effect. Thus, force yourself to procrastinate.

Once again, let me stress that you can make these tips work for you best once you have made some progress at developing an anti-procrastination philosophy, but they can be used on their own, especially in the short term.

Expect and deal with backsliding

Once you have made progress at overcoming your chronic procrastination problem, will things be plain sailing from then on? I'm afraid not. Thus, it is important that you should expect some backsliding. This means that at times you will take two steps forward and one back, and at other times you will take one step forward and two back. It is important that you recognize that this is a natural part of the change process and that you refrain from awfulizing any setbacks that you may experience. Rather, it is important that you learn from these setbacks. Thus, once you begin to procrastinate again after a period of doing tasks on time (or even ahead of time), discover the reason why you have lapsed. Frequently, the reason will be the same as the reason you procrastinated in the first place, in which case you need to go back and use the methods you used to tackle this problem originally. However, sometimes the reason you have lapsed is different from the reason you procrastinated in the first place. In this case, you need to identify the conditions that you were demanding must exist before beginning the task, in the same way as you did when learning about the reasons for your original procrastination. Then, you need to identify the demanding, awfulizing, discomfort intolerance and/or self/other depreciation beliefs that you held about the relevant activating event and their healthy alternatives, and question these beliefs using the methods that I discussed earlier in this book.

Another way of dealing with backsliding is to develop a list of factors to which you are likely to respond with procrastination. These are called vulnerability factors. I recommend that you deal with these factors in advance of encountering them, in reality by using all the methods that I have discussed in this book. You will then be better prepared for when you actually encounter these factors in real life and will be less likely to procrastinate as a result.

All humans procrastinate, since this is part of the human condition. However, if you use the methods outlined in this book and commit yourself to doing so now and in the future, you will no longer have a chronic procrastination problem. If you have put into practice the ideas and methods I have outlined in this book, I hope you have found them useful. If you have read the book first and are then planning to put what you have read into practice, I'm pleased about that. One thing, though: don't wait until tomorrow before you put them into practice. Do it now!

Index

acceptance: knowing your problem 6, 88; questioning your beliefs 36–7
Adler, Alfred 22
approval-based procrastination 60–3
attack-response technique 39–42
autonomy-based procrastination: changing attitudes 76–7; feeling encroachments 75–6; restoring the balance 22
avoidance: of discomfort 21; of threat 21
awfulizing 30; anti- 33; questioning your beliefs 36; worrying 73–4

behavioural excesses 91
beliefs: acceptance 34; acting on 44–5; anti-awfulizing 33; attack–response technique 39–42; awfulizing 30; comfort and discomfort 26–8, 30–1, 33–4, 64–6; depreciation 31–2; distorted inferences 92–4; emotive imagery technique 42–4; full preferences 32–3, 37–8; healthy 32–4, 35–9; questioning your own 35–8, 50–1; rigid demands 30; strengthening 39–44; unhealthy 29–32, 35–8

comfort and discomfort: beliefs 26–8, 30–1, 33–4, 36, 64–6; boredom 90–1; demanding quick solutions and instant achievements 68–9; distractions/instant gratification 67–8; hoping others will do tasks 23; inertia 66–7; mood-dominated action 60–72; rewards and punishments 96–7; waiting for effortless activity 69
commitment 6; to others 4–5; over-commitment 24, 81
confidence: worrying 73–4
cost-benefit analysis 7–15, 78
crisis-based procrastination 19–20, 78–9

delegation 50, 52
demands 30; questioning your beliefs 36, 37–8; quick solutions and instant achievements 68–9
depreciation 31–2
distractions and instant gratification 67–8, 90
Dryden, Windy: *How To Accept Yourself* 76; *Overcoming Guilt* 52, 57; *Ten Steps to Positive Living* 62, 94

Ellis, Dr Albert 29, 30, 91–2